MARIY

THE MUSLIM (M)OTHER

Social and Political Commentary On Contemporary Muslim Motherhood

The Muslim (M)other: Social and Political Commentary on Contemporary Muslim Motherhood

First published in England by Kube Publishing Ltd
Markfield Conference Centre Ratby Lane,
Markfield Leicestershire,
LE67 9SY United Kingdom
Tel: +44 (0) 1530 249230
Website: www.kubepublishing.com
Email: info@kubepublishing.com

© Mariya Bint Rehan 2025
All Rights Reserved. 1st impression, 2025

The right of Mariya Bint Rehan to be identified as the author of this work has been asserted by her in accordance with the Copyright, Design and Patent Act 1988. Cataloguing-in-Publication Data is available from the British Library.

ISBN 978-1-84774-249-0 Paperback
eISBN 978-1-84774-250-6 Ebook

Editor: Suma Din
Cover design and typesetting: Afreen Fazil (Jaryah Studio)

Image credits: Page 149 top row © Shadi Ghadirian, Page 149 bottom row © instragram Mouslamrabat, Page 150 © X (twitter) Europeinvasionn (account now closed), Page 151 © Instragram Future Bedouin, Dome of the Rock, Jerusalem

Printed by: ELMA Basim, Turkey.

CONTENTS

Preface   3

1. The Personal: Motherhood and The Self   9
- Mothering in the self   13
- The 'B' word   15
- Beauty and the Muslim   19
- Breaking whose stereotype?   28
- The paradox of motherhood and rediscovering yourself   34
- Realigning   39
- Truth and beauty   45
- Crossing and consolidating the ultimate borders of self   48

2. The Digital: Mothering in the Socials   55
- The Global Village   61
- Socially Not-working   71
- Mirror, mirror, on the wall…   82
- Memeification and a new social refrain   89
- Mothering in the many and everyday   95
- Motherhood as the opposite of our social-media world   101
- New frontiers   108

3. The Political: The Muslim (M)Other — 115
Once upon a time… — 118
The Muslim as Monster — 124
Human Rights, Muslims Wrong — 137
The visual standard of being Muslim — 141
The paradox of punishing Muslims for agency — 152
How the Muslim Mother is framed — 157
How we perceive ourselves as Muslim Mothers — 176
How we parent as Muslim Other — 185
Living beyond binaries — 202

4. The Cultural: PropaGender and Culturing the Muslim Mother — 211
Not MINC-ing words — 221
Our own internal algorithm — 232
Girl power? — 240
Old misogyny in Muslim Cultures — 246
Out of the Matrix… — 256
…Into the fire — 261
Introducing…the TradWife — 264
Opposing one thing does not mean endorsing its opposite — 268
Meet the Muslimah Boss — 272
An end to duality — 275
A possible solution? — 282

Postscript — 285

Acknowledgements — 295

Endnotes — 299

PREFACE

Those staid, heavy-aired and stiflingly long Sunday's when you're left to occupy the children outside of the reassuring predictability of weekday routine. The frequent, darting glances at the clock, prompting silent, internal machinations; a maternal algebra of : effort ÷ time (over quality x practicality). The passive structuring of that drawn out yawn of the day which sits unceremoniously at the final curtain between now and tomorrow. I absent mindedly nudge a discarded toy against the fibre of the multicoloured play rug with the corner of my foot, the juddering motion it creates is strangely satisfying. From the peripheries of my wandering vision, I see those all too familiar eyes, peeping out from under a heavy fringe, as my daughter stops in front of her bedroom mirror to glance at the reflection peering back at her with equal wonder.

I realise there and then, with lightening intensity, as I watch her curiosity unfold in the mirror, that there are multiple layers that will mediate the reflection that she sees and the configuration that looks back at her. For looking isn't a simple or transparent act. It's deceivingly complex, both as an action and an impression. The very performance of looking is an active one, it seeks something – reassurance, familiarity, delight, pleasure. It longs for that requited relationship. It doesn't exist without that reciprocity of subject. And the very way that subject – the visual stimuli – is internalised, mentally compartmentalised, embedded and extracted as knowledge in the hive of our perception is itself vulnerable to the multiple influences that order our thinking. That shape our very understanding and relationship with reality.

Our impression of ourselves, of others, of our place in this plain of existence is constricted by the multiple, invisible forces that tug, push, expand and constrict it. We are all always absorbing – taking in the tiny modicums of meaning that constitute the world around us in all of its moral dissymmetry – forming an impression of reality based on what's visually and ideologically available to us in our perceivable surroundings. We are constantly co-ordinating ourselves against this visual and ideological backdrop too. Very often it is hard to tell who is the active participant in the innocuous deed of 'looking' – the one that looks or the environment that stares back. Who deems and perceives who? And which party labels and defines the other..?

There are many moments that have cast and dyed me as a mother to young children, that have snowballed into the person I am today. This realisation sits as the very centre of them. In many ways it was also like holding a mirror up to myself, as a Muslim woman living and parenting in a world that often delegitimises Islam and Muslim mothers. That prickly and disconcerting realisation – that the world around my daughter would seek to define her according to its own values, colour the very impression she would have of herself according to social whims – felt like an overbearing weight. A responsibility so heavy it jogged me out of that moment of dispassion and idleness, and awoke me to a new dimension of parenting. Between me and my mirror, and my daughters and hers, is a marathon of experience that has altered the way that I look at myself. My experience, growing and perceiving that changing reflection, is what moves me to ensure hers is left pure and untainted.

There is an enduring myth surrounding parenting more generally that itself mirrors the multiple contradictions amongst which we mother. That sometimes bohemian shaped assertion that to allow your child to be "free", live unhindered by your own input, is the most natural way to parent. That the words 'natural' and 'parent' sit so unquestioningly beside each other is itself telling, and the idea that our children could be born into a vacuum or wilderness free from any kind of humanly inhibiting influence – patently false. What we neglect to acknowledge is that *both* our children and ourselves are parented by the wider culture in which we live. We, as grown, fully matured adults are swayed by the rhythms and beats of our lived environment – are persuaded which way to colour our hair, clothe and present ourselves. To presume our children are untainted by those very impulses that govern us is perhaps a little wishful. To assume we ourselves will always be the only modifying, or potentially negative, current in the waters that shape them – definitely naive. Islam hints against these delusions through its very essence – it is a decisive and affirmative way of life, a discipline which demands more from us than just our latent and passive selves, carried pliantly by the ebbs and flows of popular opinion.

And this is *not* the oft-shared story about the questionable, searching tentacles of a secular world, ready to corrupt the Muslim child. That is too black and white a fable for a world that is often mired in grey. And this binary tale itself, that we clutch onto in defensive reassurance, also exposes how blinkered our perception is by a wider narrative that doesn't belong to us. Rather, the essays you are about to read are an excavation of the environment in which we parent, as digital citizens often in secular societies, and how that impresses so intimately upon us as Muslim mums in sometimes "negative", sometimes "positive", almost always invisible ways. While that seemingly neutral canvas of space and time that we parent against may seem a negligible consideration in our broader journey as women who mother, it is the quietly humming engine upon which we gear ourselves, which we build and develop relationships with our children – that secretly motivates so much of our actions and values.

A modern parenting idiom that is more reflective of an untold truth, that so many of us carry with us, is to be mindful of the fact that our own voice becomes our child's internal voice. What greater lore for mothering is there; the idea that our rhetorical patterns traverse into and paint our children's internal walls – that this delicately invasive link is itself a single loop in an interconnected chain of history and tradition made up of mostly voiceless echoes. That this whispering fabric of language links us from one generation to the next, resonating across decades of time and geography to connect us indefinitely. A formless, tacit tradition that's indiscernible to the world at large but that we carry in our very beings. When we are so beholden to societal and cultural trends, what tones does the heatmap for this amorphous, engulfing cloud of language take? If our values become a kind of measure – negative or positive – for where our children place merit, then what do we need to deconstruct within ourselves?

In order for our children to look back at themselves, and *not* see a face they critique, a social standing they wish to elevate at the expense of others, a Muslim identity they may secretly revile, or a gender dynamic that isn't conducive to them, we need to be more cognisant of all those mediating layers that stand between them and their reflection, and us and ours.

That is, we need to be aware of the personal, social, digital, political and cultural nuances of being a Muslim mum.

CHAPTER 1

THE PERSONAL: MOTHERHOOD AND THE SELF

*And I (*Allāh*) created not the jinns and humans except they should worship Me (Alone). (Al-Dhariyat 51:56)*

Motherhood disrupts the very borders of self. The way we see, understand and experience our very selves is irreparably changed. From the physical experience of internalising and externalising another human being, to how the intimate chambers of our thoughts are shaped by their presence – how our outer boundaries become more blurred and our inner shape more porous due to this expansive care, consideration and emotional stake in another human life.

When Allāh allows us to be conduits to life we are invited to reevaluate that life. In the same way that we know a child's consciousness and sense of self is formed as they grow and develop – the very act of bringing that child into the world, that Allāh allows us to facilitate, irreversibly progresses our fundamental notions of the self; it's aim, purpose and orientation. What are the building blocks of human existence – what gives us worth, meaning, value, how do we ultimately define and measure ourselves?

Through motherhood and this fundamental obscuring of margins, Allāh gives us this unique vantage on the frontiers of existence – we teeter on those boundaries of being and not being, the material of our worldly existence and the immaterial matter of the human soul, the expressible and inexpressible.

In fact, Allāh fashioned that first bond with our as yet non-verbal baby as an unspoken one – a testament to the strength of the relationship between mother and child is that it is amongst the strongest we have, despite it being starved of the textile of language. This early, non-verbal phase in our relationship with our children sets the precedent for a connection which exceeds our linguistic selves too. While we often try to fashion language to relay this intimate and human experience, there are some experiences that language simply doesn't have the elasticity to bear. The emotional, physical and spiritual terrain of motherhood is one of those few human phenomena that words simply don't do justice to.

This tool of language which Allāh has blessed Adam with, to communicate and relate to others, is insufficient for an act which we carry so deeply in ourselves – an act which is not always relatable or communicable; the semiotics of motherhood exists in our bones. This is why it will often leave you tongue-tied in frustration, speechless in awe, and utterly consumed. On an entirely flippant note, it will leave your eyebrows doing much of the heavy lifting of parenting...

Yet here I am writing, and here you are reading, a book that tries to conceptualise the act of mothering. This is because motherhood continues to fascinate us, continues to have us reaching for the cloak of language to help us to give it a semblance of order and to bring it reluctantly into the rational domain of dialect. It is also because as Muslims who are blessed with the compass of truth, and clarity of purpose, motherhood has added significance to us both personally in how it anchors our lives, and more widely in our sense of social formation. It forms the beginning of every single one of us, the making of many of us, and remains an integral structural feature of the ummah.

And while it goes without saying that motherhood does not define us as believers, nor that we can't be believing or fulfilled without it, for those of us for whom Allāh has chosen this path, there is no denying not only that it plays a crucial role in our being, but that it also has the potential to fortify our faith.

Though we come to it from a full spectrum of positions – as professionals, wayfarers, whimsical, purposeful, young, old, organised or haphazard, we are all using Islam – the arbiter of meaning – as the constellation to guide us through this wholly sublime experience. We may have become mothers in wildly different circumstances, but the universal truth remains that Allāh has given this experience to us all as an opportunity to refine ourselves as believers, and to leave a religious legacy that will itself disrupt temporal borders – and stand as a testament for us in this life and the next. To put a flag in the sand of time, and create a well of *barakat* [1] that might wait for us on the other side. And with this experience, He grants us the irrepressible love and joy that comes with motherhood too. It is entirely singular in its mercy and blessing.

Mothering in the self

So how do we reconcile this life – and after-life – , altering event of becoming a mother, and allow it to bring out the best in us as believers and enrich our lives more generally? How do we as Muslim women, alter within ourselves once we have the added appendage of other, dependent human souls. What does it mean to be a Muslim and a mother? While we have many religious texts that frame and conceptualise this, what is the social,

---

[1] Increasing of Allāh's blessings

political and cultural reality in which Muslim mums are navigating these truths?

The fact is, despite it being one of the most intimate and personal experiences, we are not mothering in a vacuum – as personal as motherhood is, our outer boundaries of self are in friction with the exterior environment we live in. As Muslim women, the external climate and internal tension that we face today are unique. We are both blessed because we have this priceless blueprint by which to be our best selves, and uniquely challenged in how far this blueprint often contradicts a wider capitalist structure for which everything has a base value. As Muslims for whom the measure of the immaterial *barakat* shapes our worldly objectives, we are often at total odds with a system for which materiality dictates.

If, when becoming mothers, we are tasked with reconfiguring our sense of what brings value to us and our beings, and we understand that 'value' itself is perverted by capitalist sensibility, then we are in many ways starting all over again. For this reason, and many more, motherhood involves a lot of unlearning. And it all starts with the self. Because the one common, personal element that we face in this other hood of parenting is a ground swell of change in self and public perception.

The boundaries that define us personally and socially are contested conceptually too. We need to understand the climate in which our original selves are rooted and formed in order to begin to unpack our sense of self-meaning. While many of us have used different measures to value ourselves, attribute self-worth, centre our sense of identity and give us esteem and purpose, inevitably motherhood will disorder that. It will morph both the mirror through which we see ourselves, the window through which we see and categorise the world, and how that world looks back and classifies us too.

The 'B' word

And while I would love to write about Muslim motherhood without mentioning the 'B' word – the fact is it would be disingenuous to do so. The hegemonic notion of 'beauty' will always wrestle for control of the female narrative, and our own personal interests and energy. Uniquely, this is irrespective of faith, background or culture. The inescapable truth is, we live in a world that judges women entirely on their market value; in how they present their superficial surface to the external, watchful world. This is almost always either celebrated as a form of liberation or disguised as something more meaningful. And of course, it is neither. The beauty industry, both the landscape of narrative it promotes, and the components of language that prop it up, are inextricably linked to the idea of female liberation. To the point that the words we, as individual and collective women, tether ourselves to – that we think and conceive of ourselves in – are addled by a value system dictated by commercialism. We must value a 'fierceness' and that 'fierceness' must be construed in how we present ourselves externally. Women must always have an agency that is in bondage to male desire – under the pretence of benefitting ourselves. Thinness, for example, is perennially idealised in post-industrial societies where food is no longer a scarcity, as a disciplining force against women. While this language – and its values – will shift according to time, to remain relevant and profitable – more recently presenting themselves under the 'wellness' diction or body positivity – the tyrannising impact of them remains the same; beauty wields so much power over us, we are forever contorting our bodies and faces to suit changing ideals. And obviously, the external presentation of these evolving fashions is always rooted in men's interests.

'Choice feminism' has, of course, convinced us that the decisions we make are entirely free from the suffocating influence of social expectations and norms, and therefore anything we do within the context of that choice is liberating, irrespective of where the roots of those decisions lie, and who they benefit or damage. When we see a barefaced women – without the cosmetic flourishes that are in themselves designed to appeal to men; the base that is supposed to conceal signs of 'imperfection' and aging, the blush and lipstick that is designed to make us look like we have a very *specific* rush of blood to the face – it is an assault to our very senses. This is despite a man's undressed face being considered objectively public-worthy. We have been trained on an intimate, sensory level, to visually expect a certain male-defined standard of women to such an extent that it's impaired our very impulsive sense of sight.

The link between perceived female liberty and the paraphernalia of the beauty industry means that to even criticise beauty standards, the multi-billion dollar industry that upholds it, or the eternal quest for the illusive prize of being seen as 'beautiful', is deemed anti-woman, regressive, prudish and punitive. All those things Muslim women in particular are programmed to eschew as part of our fundamental identity. That stereotype we are supposed to sacrifice our entire being into dismantling (more on which, later…). This means we often cannot perceive of our worth outside of what's socially dictated to us through this paradigm of beauty. The entire concept of women's value outside of superficial measures of beauty is like a chimera to us – entirely inconceivable.

As Muslims for whom femininity is far weightier and more intrinsically linked to a deeper worth, the change of self-perception we experience when we become mothers presents a whole new rainbow of emotions and feelings. Going from understanding within you that as a woman, you have a unique and substantive worth, to actualising some of that Islamic worth in bringing new life to bear, is sobering to say the least. Crossing that border from being someone whose experience is one in which perception dictates all, to the territory of motherhood in which we are so consumed by an unperceiving, tiny little being, that demands more of you, is life altering.

Undoubtedly, we are all influenced by the broader social structures that impede and shape our personal interests and motivated behaviours – our sense of self identity – as Muslims who understand the intrinsic value of life, motherhood can aid us in reordering that sense of identity. Though we may know, and pay lip service to the idea, that we are more than just mere objects as women, the fact remains that our sentiments and inclinations as social animals are dictated by subliminal impulses not always obvious to us. We will inevitably be drawn towards certain things because we are socially programmed to conform to specific ideals and values, on a subconscious level. This is one of the most useful things you can learn as a parent – both in understanding yourself as a mum and in helping your child to do the same. As humans we have an undeniable mimetic desire; an obsession with being 'normal'. For Muslim women the stakes of that 'normal' are so much greater, they dictate our sense of legitimacy in a world that undermines it constantly. We will gravitate towards wanting to be 'beautiful' in how that's defined in any given time, despite understanding this irresistible force is not conducive to our sense of self.

Beauty and the Muslim

While Islam has protected women from the denigration that comes from being reduced to the most superficial of traits, the advent of social media and the coining of the Muslim pound has meant that the hijab has, for most of our adult life, been consumed by the machine of capital, and commodified and fetishised in the same way as any beauty-aid.

Tellingly, hijab itself is only celebrated when it is an accessory to beauty and being seen. We witness this both in the loudly celebrated online Muslim influencer sphere, but also in the various instances it is donned by non-Muslim women on red carpets and fashion events, in supposedly subversive fashion choices, which act as a kind of Muslim cosplay in which non-Muslim women are borrowing from the 'controversy' of the veil, but using it to make a statement about how they escape such restrictions to beauty. In the latter instance, hijab and modesty is effectively applauded for its objectification of women, the inverse of its purpose in Islam. When the world's most famous and displayed women cover themselves in modest-adjacent clothing, or headdresses, at Met Gala's and red carpet events, it is designed to be worn in a flippant show of wealth, fortune and their own exclusivity; the point here is that it's disposable and superfluous. And this shallow pretension is held in awe and reverence by a wider culture that denigrates any sense of faith and humility that might underpin its practical purpose.

Hijab within a faith context, worn entirely for the sake of Allāh with practical and spiritual intent, when it promotes modesty and disrupts optical availability to men, is conversely deemed dangerous and an affront to liberal sensibilities. It is that pure faith-intention alone, the volition and agency that sits beneath it, that some secular societies view with such aversion. Laughably, this invisible, intangible quality of faith is seen as hazardous, still, over 1400 years after it was first perceived to be so. Increasingly draconian policies across Europe, policing Muslim women's hijab and modesty, attests to this. Ironically in France, we have had Muslim women arrested for their choice of hijab on the beach, while non-Muslim celebrities are simultaneously celebrated for covering their face and bodies in seemingly rebellious and edgy style choices in high-fashion contexts.

The profitable dimension of hijab and modesty, which we see both here in celebrity fashion empires, and from many Muslim social media personalities, is also applauded because it is compatible with commercially-driven, mainstream sentiment. Hijab and modesty are accepted when they are part of lucrative trends, to line the pockets of fashion and beauty giants, and not with a kind of ethical intent which makes them inherently unprofitable. Hijab and modesty are only celebrated when they are co-opted into capitalist systems. The earnestness, sincerity and pure endeavour of faith more broadly – and the act of modesty in particular – are unwelcome and deemed with abject hostility precisely because they are a threat to profit. The idea that Islam is dangerous to the rich and powerful is a throughline in history which dates back to the time of the Prophet ﷺ himself; where it was the upper echelons of Quraish, those most wealthy and influential, who objected so vehemently to *laa illaha illalah* [2].

With studies in America demonstrating that over 80 percent of purchases, and purchase influence, are made by women, it is clear that there is a lot at stake financially, when women are not enslaved to the whims of fashion and beauty industries.[i] And we are only now seeing think pieces on how this is damaging to women because of how newer social media platforms are accelerating the cyclical trends that make beauty corporations so rich. Invasive cosmetic procedures and enhancements trending on TikTok – which are on a single-minded mission to fault-find women's bodies so that they are in a position to prescribe a magical, money-making, cure – have shone a blue light on the predatory nature of the beauty industry and its threat to true female liberation. It's the "hip dips", the buccal fat, or the thigh gaps we need to metamorphose our bodies in and out of – the

---

[2] The declaration of Islamic faith; there is no god worthy of worship, except Allāh

internet has gifted us a whole new punishing vernacular with which to find deficiencies in our over scrutinised and underappreciated bodies. It's a dialect that encourages us to dissociate from our very bodies, and be more visually submissive. And naturally, the language we forge through generational slang as a result, is a reflection of this. During the Millennial era of youth, when heroine chic and rake-like appearances were most desired, our complimentary slang evolved from 'sick' to this current stage of Gen Z primacy, where 'thick', more curvaceous ideals pervade, when we are now 'eating and leaving no crumbs.' Both iterations of these beauty standards – thin and disappearing and impossibly curvaceous – are equally punishing and require painful sacrifices from women. Then, and now, they are presented to us unquestionably as forms of liberation and the key to our happiness.

And so, whether it's based on YouTube's retro-hijab-tutorial era or more recent TikTok soft-girl or girlbossing your way through life, or the other various aestheticised social media trends, Muslim women have been programmed still to act and perceive ourselves in ways that will benefit male desire. This conflating of female independence and liberation with beauty and desirability is all the more complicated for Muslim women because in a world that equates women's worth to their visual acquiescence and optical availability, we will always fall short of 'womanhood' itself. Muslim women simply do not fit the conceptual bracket of femininity as it is understood by a wider system that reduces it to shallow characteristics. If womanhood as it is socially constructed involves a very particular and loud projection of beauty and sexuality, then many Muslim women simply aren't perceived as being 'women'. Modesty, and the act of being "unseen" is an affront to modern standards of femininity. And we know historically that there are cultural connotations to how Muslim women resisted visual colonisation through this radical act of covering. What happens to the Muslim female psyche, as women who have a natural affinity to our femininity, is that we often subconsciously migrate towards culturally accepted standards of femininity to fulfil that innate need to be deemed and to deem ourselves 'feminine'.

The visual norms we currently inhabit mean that being seen to *want* to be beautiful – investing in the idea that being so visibly conformist is being worthy, to commit yourself to a visual standard which puts a worth on trying to achieve desirability – is a social signal to femininity as it is culturally understood. It's being part of the Club of Woman™ as "woman" is culturally coded. For Muslim women, entry into this club not only grants them entry into womanhood, but humanhood too. The Muslim identity is continually dehumanised, alienised and aberrated, and to visibly and symbolically denounce our claim to desire beauty means we are further down the rungs of a standard which ranks humanity according to superficial traits. For Muslim women to try to claw back some sense of being acknowledged, seen, humanised, we are forced to climb this ladder of acceptability through a visual code which rewards visual acts of submission. Beautification and the act of seeking to be desirable is one way to tell the world we are human, it's one way of gleaning a sense of belonging. This is why, though the tool of beauty is used to subdue women across all races and creeds, for Muslim woman in particular, it is far more punishing. As beauty, or our visible endeavour towards it, is presented as a gateway to far more than just being desirable. It's a means by which we are seen as human.

We belong, and are immersed in, a visual language that we are unwilling participants in. In a world where commodity reigns and surface and appearance is everything, we unknowingly become preoccupied with being consumable. The act of conforming visually, of paying symbolic credence to a value system which grades women according to how much they are willing to commit to a beauty standard, gives us a false sense of agency – it gives us the untrue impression that we are in control of how we are visually consumed and culturally catalogued. A false idea that we are not being carried by a wave of conformity, in the sea of submission. The visual training we receive, and the symbolic language we speak, is something we often unconsciously submit to.

When actually, to be purposeful and conscious of our visual landscape and the place we inhabit in it, is actually where empowerment lies. Yet this line of Islamic reasoning, and the way we read and understand the language that shapes it, is inherently unpopular and deemed intrinsically dated because we read femininity as proximity to beauty. In a world that worships the novel, which is shaped by the cyclical trends of fashion, there are no two worse things than being dated and unfashionable. This reading of femininity warps our fundamental understanding of ourselves, our sex, and our faith. But there is a beauty in accepting yourself outside of the constraints of surveillance capitalism's monopoly of what it means to be female. And there is both happiness and lightness in keeping your beauty to yourself, and in valuing that self, outside the literal and metaphorical filters that dictate our sense of worth.

In a world of Only Fans, ubiquitous cosmetic enhancement and a titanic beauty industry, the act of covering, and modesty as an endeavour, remains radical in the most unparalleled of ways. When we are encouraged to share, reveal our inner and outer world, the quiet act of keeping something to yourself will always defy understanding. As women are encouraged to dress, redress, shape and reshape themselves in line with a standard that revolves around the male vantage, the hijab and niqab will always remain a thing of curiosity and confusion, especially to a wider world which seeks to put a price tag on everything.

In the twilight of 'diversity, equity and inclusion' culture, many of us have been fed a cultural diet which privileges a very singular idea of representation. In reality, the fashion and beauty industry attest to the fact that there is very little Muslim women have gained from the zeitgeist of 'representation'. Muslim women are still scapegoated culturally and politically in the West, and attitudes and laws concerning the hijab appear to be regressing in much of the world. Similarly, high profile Muslim women in entertainment and media have made little material difference to the true advancement of Muslim women in Western countries as a whole, beyond this commercialisation and a shallow, cultural nod in our direction. Inclusivity of visibly Muslim women by and large is a grand-scale equivalent of a condescending pat on the head. There appears to be very little effort to meaningfully engage with the purpose or value of hijab as an expression of faith, in order to tackle the bigotries that society possesses. Rather, mainstream efforts merely celebrate their own supposed depth in acknowledging and tolerating it. It is a hollow, self-congratulatory attempt at equity which focuses on majority comfort rather than 'minority' inclusion, and speaks of a cultural hubris and naval gazing that is a real impediment to true inclusion, whatever that might look like.

Indeed, Islam is only accepted of us when it sits, tokenistic, in the background of our existence, barely in view, like a silent and docile pet. When it is a driver of our actions and practical and purposeful in intent, it becomes an impediment – an inconvenient reminder to the wider world of a life beyond the shiny and profane.

Breaking whose stereotype?

As Muslim women, our very claim to femininity is also obscured through a narrative which pervades public thought and opinion – and which impacts us as mums so acutely; the 'breaking the stereotype' trope. It becomes incumbent upon us to prove ourselves by performing to shatter historical, racist assumptions, that never belonged to us or our religious tradition in the first place. Muslim women are tasked with proving ourselves against a figment of racist imagination; we must NOT be the submissive wife, the obedient daughter, or the self-sacrificing mum. All roles which were created by the West to justify military, cultural and imperial dominance – the literature, arts and media concerning Muslim women in Afghanistan pays testament to this. In this era of Islamophobia, we are expected to perform against these older racist labels, by embracing the newer, shinier ones; it's not Racism, it's Diet Racism.

Muslim women in times of war and peace are encouraged to engage in a self-contorting insanity to create a circus whose sole purpose is to satisfy a secular gaze which is itself wrestling with its own conscience. We must be skateboard wielding, independent, career-pursuing women. And, of course, the arts and corporate advertising's obsession with Muslim women on wheels needs to be unpacked for everybody's well-being. If you are intent on getting misty eyed and self-fawning about a supposedly edgy ideal you feel your culture has proffered to a class of women

– because you have dehumanised them so much their very existence outside of the stereotypes you shoehorn them into appears revelatory to you – then really the call may be coming from inside the house.

This expectation to succumb to another more current fruit of racist thinking, this time by eschewing the historical seeds that bore it, is nothing more than a waste of time and a distraction. The idea that Muslim women must performatively demonstrate they are 'bold', 'intelligent', 'independent' or anything else on the list of benign adjectives, exposes the limitations of both mainstream assumptions of Muslim women and their impoverished perceptions of those very traits in themselves. Boldness need not be expressed through a shade of lipstick, and intelligence should not have to manifest itself in terms of our salaried worth. This is not our cultural baggage and we don't need to take it on as a barometer of our success; our lives, values and most importantly, our religion, are not beholden to these ideas. Our liberation comes from refusing to pander to the limitations of racist and colonialist minds.

Ultimately, the truth remains, even when we adopt what are perceived as secular constructs of femininity, it is not enough to initiate us into the private sorority of womanhood, as is evident in the case of Algerian boxer Imane Khelif, and the diabolical gender row during the 2024 Paris Olympics.[ii] On the surface, Khelif is the embodiment of liberalism and its pet, corporate media's, dream; a fiercely strong, fighting, Muslim woman – shattering every perceivable stereotype and uninhibited by the constraints of 'Islamism'. The corporate logo is poised and ready to take centre stage in her success. Yet despite being 'liberated' according to these ideals, she was deemed a threat to the very notion of 'womanhood' – her identity as Muslim, and her opposer's identity as European, was integral to this demonisation. That is – when a Muslim woman meets those standards so graciously set out for us by secular culture – those very standards are then weaponised against us, and considered a threat to womanhood itself. Underscoring this is the idea that modern notions of femininity very much exclude the Muslim woman, by default, herself – irrespective of what cultural caveat or secular appendage we attach to our very beings.

The "Breaking the Stereotype" narrative that Muslims become unwittingly enmeshed in means we are afforded humanity through our adjacency to liberal notions of femininity. Our apparent value comes from being conceptually intelligible to others. We are understood – and culturally seen – if we invest our identity into massaging the liberal ego. As Muslim women, we are not obliged to alter our very being for others' visual or intellectual consumption. The truth is Muslim women, of their own accord, can and will fit on a more nuanced spectrum which will incorporate some of these arbitrary rankings of worth. Surprisingly, we are not 2D cut-out figures in a wider game of social expectations.

The male gaze, which directs popular notions of femininity, is inherently lazy, it seeks a kind of visual gratification that serves its interests and desires. The hijab, and modesty, subverts and desists that gaze. This has created a visual culture whereby as Muslim women, we often adopt the practicality of hijab and modesty, but are simultaneously labouring to ensure we are culturally catalogued and visually indexed in a way that is non-threatening and pacifying to the wider world. Often, in the way we alter our public-facing selves to appease mainstream notions of beauty, we are honing and adjusting that unsought spectatorship back onto us.

And of course, motherhood is one of the primary things we as Muslim women must qualify through other means, to appear meaningful to the world. This constant din of public discourse and thought, that we see repeated in the highest of Government offices, and on an everyday level on the street – that Muslim women are only good for being mothers and being a mother is only good for the passive, empty symbol of the Muslim woman. Both 'Muslimness' and the symbol of 'mum' are pulled down and further denigrated by this associative label. It asserts a normative ideal that, given the weight of stereotype we carry, we must be more than *just* a mum, and that we might achieve something with some semblance of remarkable if we are appendaged with more than just 'mum'. As though that three letter, unassuming and everyday English word doesn't encompass, and isn't encompassed by, so much of what is meaningful to ourselves and society at large. As though it isn't the first word that many of us form, a primary element of our language, identity and thinking – the first notion of love, comfort, warmth, happiness and stability most of us encounter; all uncommodifiable, intangible things that materialist culture glitches in response to. Undoubtedly, Muslim women can and will be more than what we identify as 'mothers' because we are (massive shock and true horror…) whole humans – slaves of Allāh. But the fact remains, this identity of the Muslim mum is the ultimate pigeonhole we are all told implicitly and explicitly by the world at large, that we *must*, at all cost, be more than and reach further beyond. Often, unsurprisingly, the more contrasting to the role of 'mother' we assume, the more social advantage we accrue. Roles that are as far away from the private, non-profitable, nurturing, and invisible have more social currency, especially for Muslim women. This creates a strange and congratulatory pride that we all silently carry in us, for being as remote to 'motherly' as we can be. As though we carry the shame of being a 'mother' in our most unconscious selves.

The pressure to prove ourselves according to other people's prejudice is not something any woman should take upon themselves for the sheer futility of it. This doesn't mean that the Muslim mum should 'restrict' herself to motherhood – but that our realities and identities should never be in submission OR defiance to any ridiculous, recurrent man-made trends and values. Despite ad agencies across the globe achieving a sense of marketing-euphoria in feeling they've invented the (Muslim) wheel…

The paradox of motherhood and rediscovering yourself

All factors considered, as women you will, therefore, inevitably feel a different kind of way once the label 'mother' is attached so visibly (and audibly…) to your being. Many mums will articulate this as feeling 'frumpy', 'past it', 'over the hill' and so on… because the social semiology of womanhood is cruel and punishing… What this actually means is the ground beneath you has shifted – and your social standing is changing. You will most likely feel this in the most visceral of ways because it's something that society manufactures below the realms of what's perceptible – it's like a silent engine on which we operate, but don't acknowledge. Society places a strange contradictory value on a woman's ability to conceive. It is both desirable and punishable. In fact, the beauty industry – and the highly coveted value of being 'pretty' – is entirely predisposed upon perceived fertility. Women have been socially trained to want to be desirable – a desirability that is both implicitly and explicitly linked to perceived fertility, affability, and docility. And so, socially, the notion of youth, beauty and the idea of fertility on which it is based, is considered advantageous, but the physical act of being a mother will also make you as an individual woman feel hugely looked down upon by that same standard. In one of society's cruellest acts, it frames and perceives women as a depleting stock, while it extends the opposite grace towards men. A woman's value is apparently cheapened as she ages due to this perception of compromised or reduced fertility, while male capital increases owing to a higher earning power as they age. This cultural cipher, encrypted in our social DNA, is something we come to a kind of sobering realisation of as we age. It creates a kind of fist-to-the-world abandon in many of us, that we feel most around the time of having children, when our biology understands this entirely socially construed injustice most acutely.

Going from someone who is desirable because of their potential to have children, to undesirable because they have a child, overnight, pretty much sums up this contradictory social value of motherhood. If a woman's worth is placed on her availability to men, then motherhood signals an end to that kind of openness and availability. It is almost as if society has utilised your worth – and so you are chewed up and spat out according to this social function by which you were once deemed valuable. Being a mum will take you out of that bracket of girlishness – ready, available, and noticeable – and on to new plains – locked down, otherwise occupied, unavailable and invisible – according to a value system governed by male interests.

Own ~ and I cannot stress this enough ~ it.

Being dislodged from this value system can allow us to re-understand ourselves. As Muslim women who are personally and spiritually invested in a doctrine which has always allowed us to perceive our worth *beyond* the measure of beauty, sexuality and reproductive capacity, it can be the beginning of a different kind of emancipation. It is a moment of epiphany, falling back into your innate sense of self. As women living amongst a visual and cultural landscape that upholds the 'beauty myth', our default sense of self is intimately tied to this currency of 'girlhood', the only way we can perceive and measure ourselves is against this very specific notion of femininity, and it may cause a kind of social vertigo to be uncoupled from it. But we often do not realise we are prisoners to something until we are free – however unnerving that may initially feel. We are, as a culture, wed to this idea that 'authenticity' means your most embryonic or whimsical self. That to be true to oneself – and therefore valid and right – is to unquestioningly act upon instinct. This is false because our most authentic being is our fitrah –

and returning to it requires an active labour, and a decoupling from this idea that we must be loyal to an earlier sense of self – pre-baby, pre-adulthood, or pre-anything other than what we might endeavour to improve ourselves to be according to His law.

For the first time ever you are free from the social expectation, and your own obligation to it, to be 'girlish' in how that's culturally perceived – kittenish, affectated, purse-lipped and inoffensively feisty – and all the other strange and pacifying connotations we attach to female youthfulness, that have such purchase in a cultural economy designed by and for strange men. This means you can start to appreciate yourself outside of the shackles of these expectations; there is no pressure to appear in a way that adheres to any of these ridiculous, archaic and base criteria. Once you are forced to see yourself outside of that conceptual bracket, you will have the opportunity to realise yourself on your own terms, to unpick yourself from the male gaze that has dictated so much of you for so long, to understand yourself whole and untainted. It is both a liberating and unburdening feeling, and for many women it's the beginning of a journey to true self-discovery.

Realigning

If becoming a mum presents an opportunity to avoid the denigrating hurdles of beauty standards; the Muslim adaptations of it, and the stereotypes we must eschew as a result – then really it is a chance to delearn, reprogramme and rediscover the grain of your being. Your interests, talents, strengths and gifts, away from the distractions that make them seem irrelevant. Liberal and capitalist-fuelled notions of womanhood are centred on being seen – perceived as beautiful and alluring – and our preoccupation with how we are viewed means we lose sight of ourselves, and allow ourselves to be subsumed into whatever (ultimately pedestrian and anodyne…) trend of desirability that dominates our time. From pro-Anna to the Instagram face we must colour and contour ourselves into. Existing in the moment, and living to actually feel and experience, rather than just to be 'seen', are often laboured concepts for women who are socially trained to be so painfully and acutely conscious of how they are perceived.

The female psyche, as famous visual culturists explain, is divided into a 'surveyor' and the 'surveyed'[iii], and our self-policing psychology is shaped by this sport of spectatorship– we are constantly aware of how we are perceived because of the optical landscape we are drawn into. We assume within ourselves, the punishing male gaze, it enters our interior space – we are, at all times, cognisant of how we are perceived according to male interests. It appears, as Muslims, we have also internalised a kind of secular gaze by which we survey ourselves – an additional dimension to this punitive process, which means we are also weighing ourselves up, and are subliminally motivated by, secular values and thinking. These bent and warped prisms through which we order our self-perception are ultimately inhibiting and cumbersome, they represent additional, restrictive layers to our being. If motherhood is a disruption of those inner and outer boundaries, then this is something we have the opportunity to purge, to redraw ourselves on a blank canvas against new lines, with a renewed sense of value and worth.

If reaching maturity marks the beginning of our journey as women, perceiving ourselves in new ways, and inhabiting a new social space – then becoming a mother bookmarks it in many ways – it's a significant milestone which allows us to really reassess those ways we perceive ourselves. It is the beginning of a new phase in our lives and the end to potential others.

This can mean rediscovering religious tenets. Allāh has allowed us through the beauty of modesty to protect ourselves from the whimsical changes in society and fashion that would otherwise dictate our sense of self and social worth. Allāh has created woman so that she does not reduce her own worth to a meagre object, and posits value in the 'now'; the act of being, achieving, experiencing, rather than the passive act of merely being perceived – an act entirely contingent upon the surveyor and how it perceives her, and which robs her of any agency and rids her of any control. In Islam, our worth as women goes way beyond and outside of our reproductive capacity, we are believers with far more intrinsic value than our role as mothers, or as those potentially desirable to men, might give us alone. The irony of course being that popular opinion often denigrates Islam and Muslim women, wrongly, for being reduced to mere accessories to men, with the sole purpose to child rear. Islam gives us far more room to breathe and grow than the straitjackets of social expectations.

And while many of you reading this will be going through an 'ah-ha' moment – thinking this is the inevitable bit where the scolding aunty-narrative sets in, urging you to retire your lipsticks and commit to the heinous idea of being "ugly" – I want to assure you that this is actually the bit where we acknowledge that Allāh created us all beautiful, and anything extraneous to you is a distraction that plays on your most subliminal fears. It's the part where we need to recognise that any voice which enters your head telling you otherwise, certainly with as much confidence as it does, is something that needs uprooting from your internal world.

Motherhood presents us with the opportunity to realise part of ourselves outside of the lens of desirability. In this way, it provides a window to living and experiencing ourselves in the moment, not for perception and appearance alone. It's like taking off your shoes and feeling the grass beneath your feet for the first time – familiar and unfamiliar at the same time. Like listening to a voice you thought you lost. Ultimately, it can be the beginning of living your life truly for the sake of Allāh, and not those multiple invisible social forces that will dictate your actions and worth. It is centring Allāh's gaze in your life, and not the human construct of the male, or secular, gaze.

Ironically, as Muslim women, we are used to a form of female liberation which might denounce beauty ideals from a materialistic perspective, but shies away from rooting that in Islamic principles

– as though it is only worth reclaiming our lost rights and reasserting ourselves if it's based on secular notions of freedom and liberation that are intelligible to society as a whole. This means, we might be able to construe that we have gained something, and are stronger, from rebelling against beauty ideals because we understand they are restrictive to our own sense of personal agency, but we may not understand that doing that, and anything else, for the sake of Allāh alone is where our truth lies, even if it's not as edgy or aestheticiced. Our reward comes from doing things for Him who is Most Merciful - it is the most purifying intention. As Muslims in a now globalised culture, we are accustomed to speaking of our faith using borrowed language, appropriated terms, and fashionable slogans, and are therefore sometimes unable to conceive of it acutely. As an ethical system that is entirely unique in how it resists all forms of commodification, our faith – both in terms of its intricacies and broader values – is not something we will see adequate representation of in popularised culture. Therefore it is something we need to build an understanding of outside of popular sensibilities and language.

While our sense of meaning and purpose is often obscured through the white noise of social expectations, we are often oblivious to both understanding and living our lives in alignment with what we were created for. '*Insān*'[3] is connected by root to the verb '*nasiya*' which means 'to forget' in Arabic. It is part of our very nature to need to be reminded, to have to recall and reinforce the beauty of our faith and the purpose of our design. Similarly, our desired state to be in constant '*tawbah*'[4] comes from the root '*tabah*' – to come back. We are in need of constantly returning to Him, ceaselessly coming back to The Bestower, in search of His Mercy and blessings. Often, despite thinking we know, we need to be reinspired, retold and reinvigorated – we need to go back to the book of Allāh, to His Sunnah.[5]

As your child grows, and you in this new phase in your life grow too, if you listen attentively enough, you will hear that voice within you that some of us have buried for so long, reminding you to close the gap between your actions and values. To return to those moments of passion and rigour in learning and enacting your religion in earnest – because Allāh blesses us all with those beautiful highs in *imaan*[6] to leverage when

---

[3] Man
[4] Repentance
[5] Teachings, practices and examples set by the Prophet Muhammed ﷺ
[6] Faith

we are low. To embody Islam's unique focus on connecting knowledge to action, and action to intention. To implement that truth without all our interior monologue caveats that take you away from its practical, and enriching, material implications. Those that come hand in hand with Islam and in which true peace and happiness are predisposed. It's not a voice you will necessarily find echoed on social media, complemented by consumer culture, nor necessarily one that makes you feel 'seen' in a world dictated by perception and appearance. But that doesn't make it bad.

Truth and beauty

If we intend to learn from recent, tragic world events like the genocide in Gaza, that have shattered our sense of moral safety, and notions of truth and beauty, then we must acknowledge that truth itself is a discipline and not something we passively absorb from the world around us. It is a doctrine and a form of learning with fidelity to our holy text alone, and it is that faithfulness that will provide us closest to a semblance of contentment, not the currents of popular judgment which seek to shape, and reshape, our sense of self and identity according to contemporary trends in morality. In order to lead purposeful lives – anchored in meaning, and which are directional –

it's important to interrogate societal values. Truth is an active endeavour. And personal whims and the cultural norms that they uphold do not, and should not, shape our value system or the practices that emanate from them. And that applies to the truth we hold of ourselves – and how honest we are about our intentions and actions.

While the pretensions that we embodied in a world before that of October 2023 lose their shine and appeal, and the sobering cold of our current world sets in, we are reminded that Islam is the only sedimentary quality we possess. When we are witness to the transience of life, and the injustice of the world, we affirm that Islam is the only thing that has material value and weight between this fragile existence and the next, that will take us between here and the black space that separates us from the hereafter. Islam protects our minds and hearts from the heady delusions of this world, a world in which happiness is always fleeting, and which is solely a corridor to our true and eternal selves. Allāh has promised us that if we follow His words, not only will those moments of beauty in this corridor seem less ephemeral, but also that we may find hope in those instances of pain and hardship too. But most importantly, that what awaits us at the end of it, will be so beautiful and perennial, that none of that hardship will matter anymore.

This is pertinent and more obvious in motherhood because you will be modelling this life and value system so acutely to your children. If we are so influenced by those broader value systems that surround us, imagine how much the subtle hues of our inner and outer selves impress upon our children for whom we are their first and foremost teachers, trainers and models during their most impressionable years. Our development as mothers and believers will imprint upon and shape theirs. We see how our young children borrow actions, traits and characteristics from the world around them. When they are very young we glean a kind of wonderment and pleasure in tracing each of the quirks of their being to their external influences; which expression and gesture they picked up from which sibling, grandparent or uncle. As they grow they become more complex and tangled expressions of their outer environment, to the point that we cannot unpick each of the strands to attribute to its original source. Our job as mothers is to mediate that pulsating web of the external world, to understand the enmeshing strings of influence that may knot and twist beyond what we deem suitable, and tirelessly attempt to temper them through the uncompromising truth of Islam.

Crossing and consolidating the ultimate borders of self

As believing mothers who embody those borders between the material and immaterial, it should be more obvious to us the way our actions and intentions will also reverberate, crossing borders of time through generations; onwards and beyond our current plain of existence. The intrinsic and weighty value of good intentions and deeds are made most evident when we interact with the next generation, including for those of us who are directly raising them. We, on a daily basis, are witness to how this *barakat* that we seek, that sweetens our lives here and eternally, is carried through our intentions and actions. How it travels through that fourth dimension of time within our children, and the values and habits we implant in and through them. Because Islam is sent to us from The Greatest, Who created our soul, and knows our needs better than we know them ourselves, it is underpinned by a science and knowledge that He has provided us with in His infinite Mercy, to aid us to make the most out of His Mercies and maximise our happiness.

While there is now many a modern idiom from tech entrepreneurs and other men that society most adulates about how the sobering realisation of death has contributed to their achievements in life, we forget that mothers who are so instrumental in the process of life, are equally living a life-affirming consciousness that is ripe for producing success. As with many fields of science related to women, the neural changes in the maternal brain are criminally understudied – but early research suggests women get more certain and focused in their thinking when pregnant.[iv] As mums, we experience a kind of realness that brings you down to your absolute core – that grants you a perspective that is unparalleled. Allāh gives us this as an opportunity to live for the sake of Allāh alone, and to assist those most beloved to us to see the enrichment and beauty in that too.

As the days of childhood are knitted and pearled into weeks, years and decades, you will be the living embodiment of how your child will see, learn and enact their faith. You will be the constant gardener of their *imaan*. You will begin to experience time as a different medium – an inevitable force, the matter of our very being. We are ultimately an amalgamation of the deeds we accrue, and amassing those virtuous actions in all that we weather is all that really matters.

Islam is entirely consistent as a belief system – we worship Allāh through practices that dictate our day and lives; praying and fasting. And we worship Him through smaller momentary actions such as smiling when we greet someone. These smaller actions create an intricately woven and beautiful whole that's entirely aligned with our overall sense of purpose and direction. Motherhood presents you with an opportunity, in the best possible way, to sweat the small stuff and live that beautiful tapestried whole which centres Allāh, and gives you an unmatched peace and harmony. Allāh is Al-Haseeb; Ever a Careful Account Taker of all things – He keeps records of all actions and He requites them. Not a leaf falls but He knows it. How precious is this medium of time He has granted us to make the most out of all the ways we can please Him. In the same way we experience the sweetness of khushu in those moments our thoughts and actions are aligned in worship, we have the opportunity to extend that unity in how we think and live as Muslims. To align our heart, tongue, limbs and the direction of our lives – together – and experience that edifying nectar of living our fitrah as permanent architectural features that decorate our whole, full lives.

In a capitalist value system, our notion of morality mimics our economics, we are psychologically wired to treat morality like a dwindling currency. We view our goodness as a finite resource which we dish out in rations; *I've done my good deed for the day*' is not an unfamiliar phrase to many of us. Inverting this attitude that has migrated into our faith practice; to be miserly with the deeds of our heart, tongue and limbs – to begin to see life outside of the transactional prism of capitalism, to view the good as an ever increasing pool which grows as we utilise it, and to outgrow the mindset that we gain 'haram points' for committing a good deed, are all things that can only help us in the eternal and fortifying endeavour we adopt as Muslims to self-improve, grow, expand and always strive to be better. Despite the social pull to glorify sin, it is time to drop the *halal: haram*[7] ratio that we sometimes proudly brand ourselves by. This mind shift, to see Islam outside of a deficit model which frames Islamic principles as strange and lacking, a tick box exercise at the expense of 'happiness'; rather to see them as beautiful and bountiful, replete with wisdom beyond our comprehension, will inevitably plug the deficiencies in our lives. This intellectual clog in our thinking is what makes us drag our heels

---

[7] Religiously lawful: unlawful

in the quest for self-improvement, to seek the momentary comfort of familiar at the expense of the temporary discomfort that we face before we achieve moral growth.

Allāh has sent us parallels in our civilisational, social and cultural development as a people. The anthropological model of religion is the mirror opposite of what we know to be true in Islam. It asserts that man came from polytheism and refined himself into man-made monotheism through collective social and political advancements like the nation-state. In reality, we know that Allāh implanted the shahadah in our hearts, and sent us Prophets to keep us guided when we strayed. This macro model presents the micro one we need to implement in our lives, a constant returning to the truth. Islam was sent for the individual and collective benefit – that it begins with interrogating your inner most motivations is telling in itself. And that's because society has a tendency to erect and worship false idols, to be drawn towards the shiny and profane, despite the noble intention Allāh has placed in all of us. This is implicit in everything around us – be it our atavistic desire to be a slave to our impulsive whims, the grandiose origin narratives we craft about ourselves, or the cultural icons we appoint.

And so, while the personal implications of motherhood present their own opportunities to alter the borders of self and public perception, there is nothing more important than turning both inward in how you deconstruct that self, and outward to the word of Allāh in how you rebuild it. In connecting yourself to your Creator through your thoughts, intentions and actions. To leave no stone unturned in the quest for self-improvement. And of course, this extends to how we conduct ourselves as social beings too.

Ihsan[8] is a quality we should all strive towards as Muslims – it is one of our defining features as an ummah. And *ihsan* has different meanings in *shariah* – there is, of course, *ihsan* in worship – we know from the famous hadith of *Gibrael* that the highest form of worship is to worship Allāh as though you see Him, and if not, then at least to know that He can see you. But there is also the *ihsan* of kindness or doing good – and this has two branches; *ihsan* with Allāh and *ihsan* with the *khalq*.[9] As Muslims, we strive to perfect ourselves in regards to the rights we fulfil towards Allāh, but also the rights we must fulfil towards creation. In the Quran, the two most frequent acts of worship mentioned together are *salat* and

---
[8] Roughly translated to 'perfection'
[9] Creation

zakat – mirroring this dual duty to the Creator foremost, but also His creation. This begs the question, what do we need to be cognisant of, socially, as Muslim mums?

CHAPTER 2

THE DIGITAL: MOTHERING IN THE SOCIALS

> *No vision can grasp Him, but His Grasp is over all vision. He is the Most Subtle and Courteous, Well-Acquainted with all things. (Al-Anaam 6:103)*

Once you escape the restrictive net of the male gaze, it is so easy to seek that reassurance, validation and punishment elsewhere. A lot of the time women come out of the frying pan only to be consumed by the fire of the righteous Mum brigade, made angrier by the expansive black hole of the internet. There is, of course, so much value in contemporary mothering discourse – the reason online spaces for mums are such a comfort is the plethora of voices they grant us access to. There is always a baby that's lodged the same item up its nostril as yours. That shared experience and sense of connectivity is undoubtedly a blessing, but it can also be a curse, when we use it for self or public adoration or shaming.

So while you are still high on the emancipation from male expectations, do not fall so easily into the fetters of the social expectations of motherhood. Take what you can from the science, experiences, and opinions of mothering online and offline, and despite the muscle memory we have for approval seeking, resist the urge to come into a new fold of affirmation. If motherhood allows us to ground ourselves in the most fundamental way – to break down the very elements of our own sense of self-perception, self-worth and self-fulfilment – the last thing we want to do is refashion that into another model which seeks anything other than Allāh's approval. That blanket of social validation that we seek is insufficient in providing us the with the warmth that we crave.

As women, social pressure is not alien to us – as we've explored in some depth. And as Muslims who have experienced adolescence, many of us have endured the proverbial baptism of fire that constitutes being young and Muslim. Muslim adolescence is often particularly testing due to the obvious broader influences which shape our young and impressionable minds. While data shows that younger Gen Z's – the online, remote generation – adopt more socially conservative behaviours than generations that preceded them in certain ways – with sexually risky behaviour, drug taking and alcohol consumption trending downwards[v] – most Muslim mums today, who cut their adult tooth on a culture replete with vices antithetical to Islam, have internalised the notion of "sin as rite of passage". The social expectations on young people was, and still is, to engage in what Islam classes as illicit activities that act as cultural gateways to adulthood. Becoming sexually active and drinking alcohol, to name two legal examples, are considered ceremonial to maturity according to popular practice and opinion. What this unwittingly means is Islamic values and practice – the acts of abstinence, restraint and rectitude – are subconsciously infantilised according to popular thought, and this naturally shapes our own perception of Muslim maturity too. The Muslim, and Islamic culture, is perennially less than – not quite fully evolved, in a constant state of not being enough – due to a refrain from these ostensibly coming-of-age activities. This is the root of some of the adolescent embarrassment that being Muslim often carries; that in being Muslim, and embodying the characteristics of modesty, chastity and other forms of discipline, we are unknowing, inexperienced and 'childish' in nature, with all the cultural baggage and stigma that invites.

While undoubtedly Islam champions some of the implications of innocence which carry such common disapproval, the idea that supposedly verdant Muslims are morally, culturally and intellectually immature or rudimentary is nonetheless false and misleading. As are the ways those popular constructs of 'adulthood' mature into 'parenthood,' and what that means for how motherhood itself is built and idealised and projected onto concepts of Muslimness. We may be programmed to believe that certain practices that we ascribe to, as individuals and parents, are not 'normal', perhaps a little 'silly', somehow needing cultural approval and state sanction. But we cannot measure the worth of an act by how many people engage in it, and this is something we need to remind ourselves of, even in this later stage of our lives. These perceptions of 'normality' will bleed into how Muslim parents are viewed in the West and how those values we choose to share with our children are delegitimised. Muslim parents are equally widely overlooked in contemporary policy making in Western countries because they are not considered legitimate, and their views and opinions are dismissed and undermined.

If acts that are impermissible in Islamic faith are seen as a means into adulthood, then as Muslims who promote a culture that withholds from such things, our faith is deemed unnatural, subversive and objectionable. It is at best something that is paternalistically and condescendingly 'tolerated' and at worst aberrated as dangerous and a threat to our very children – who are themselves in their very nature and being, deemed suspicious too… Our faith means the very act of conceiving and raising children, and the practices we engage in, are geared towards a religious value. Against a backdrop of secularism, or anti-Muslim sentiment, this is deemed either an entirely foreign concept or it is needlessly perceived as 'dangerous' – sometimes both. The Muslim family is therefore rendered a destabilising force to the state and society at large for this reason and many more, as we shall go on to inspect when we look at the politics of Muslim motherhood in the next chapter.

Like the popular construct of the Muslim woman as "submissive" stereotype, or "fierce" counterstereotype that we examined in the previous chapter, in the debate concerning how motherhood is socially constructed in the blogosphere, Islam is entirely absent, despite prominent voices evoking Islam to justify their views and expand their audience. As we will also go on to interrogate in the final chapter on the cultural implications of Muslim motherhood, Muslim women are influencers, and influenced by, the broader cultural movements that are born on the internet. Almost always, this is using borrowed language and inherited cultural norms that are not native to our faith. The social pressures that Muslim mums are under is shaped by the global culture of the internet, and often 'Islam' is an afterthought in how this is branded to us as consumers.

But what about the social and now digital hues of Muslim motherhood?

The Global Village

The hyperconnected digital world that we now inhabit means that, where previously we may have had the village as our community – we have now extended that, and are exposed and vulnerable to, the entire human population. The surveying digital eye has permeated through our most intimate and private spaces – we have effectively domesticated the public sphere and publicised the domestic sphere, and the distinctions we place upon both are now supple and prone to movement. This means both the pressure we get from spectators of the sport – non-mums – and the intra-community issues within mum circles, are amplified. The weight of parenting norms, ideals and communities come in global volume. As the stage from which we mother, and the audience which is privy to it, has grown exponentially, so has our capacity for both validation and shame; with the web of complexity that brings to our sense of personal and social growth. When we look at what mothers gain from the village – there is the positive; support, structure, advice, care – and the negative; negative potential to shape normative behaviours, shallow and counterproductive affirmation, and false and damaging hierarchies. Both sides of this coin are magnified in the age of digital motherhood.

And these social pressures begin with the construct of the Mum herself, without any added faith value.

In fact, there are few subjects which invite such polemic response as mothering. It is an emotionally laden, high stakes area of discourse. Almost without exception, the social expectations of motherhood that we see propagated in digital spaces do not represent Islamic perspectives. They are both punitive and contradictory. You only have to look at how mothering culture online is framed to get an insight into the highly contested ways in which society, and now internet culture, label mum groups. There is a begrudging and condescending acknowledgement of what's often characterised as a 'smug' Mums-net 'cartel' culture which attracts derision – a sentiment forged from male, and often right-wing, voices and opinions – a sneering attitude which belittles our worth. Here we see mums construed as an overindulged demographic, that probably have it all too easy, and who are excessively vocal and influential; the 'Facebook Mum' pejorative. The irony being, of course, that many of these men will encourage women to adopt the role of mother to 'qualify' them, and use their right wing credentials as those who purport to privilege 'family values' to distract from their sadistic misogyny. There is also the counter idea that motherhood is passive, outdated slave labour, which emanates from female, often leftist, spaces and at its core understandably fixates on the sheer amount of solitary emotional and physical labour intrinsic to motherhood, as well as economic and social penalties women are subject to. As part of this wider sentiment, we see the focus on motherhood as a toxic domain to be avoided at all cost, and the idea that as women, we are far greater than this biological function. Both the anti-natalist trends amongst young women and pro-natalist trends and increasing social conservatism from men are interestingly attributed to a sharp decline in fertility rates in the West, owing to the higher numbers of childless women born from the mid-eighties onwards in Western countries.[vi] Motherhood, and mothers, appear to be under attack from all political directions and across genders and it is having a material impact on our lives and choices. These ideological backdrops act as touchpoints for Muslim culture, which has absorbed and adapted many of these ideas through a process of cultural osmosis.

Perhaps what epitomises this torrid discursive landscape is a September 2024 front cover of The New Yorker magazine, which tapped into this zeitgeist of conversation regarding maternal realities, and the many variables which surround it, and garnered over sixty million views and many thousands of comments on Twitter/X alone. The cover art which depicted two older women of colour child minding two young white children in a park setting, with one nanny proudly displaying to the other a picture of what appears to be her own son graduating.[vii] The cover was so culturally evocative as, as well as intimating at the geopolitical and racial nuances to mothering, it perfectly framed the modern day notion of motherhood as both luxury and exploitative labour in just one image. These two older women were adopting the 'burden' of child-rearing for those in a better economic position, and therefore were missing out on the indulgence of raising their own. The racial elements of course hint at the continued rich, predominately white outsourcing of maternal labour – including through surrogacy – from the West to the third world, which as a phenomenon itself is a minefield. But it also hinted at a deeper problem concerning the very taxing nature of mothering against a backdrop which penalises mothers. Research demonstrates that though fewer young women are choosing parenting, and though it rates decidedly lower as a personal aspiration, many see time spent with their children as a more enriching or 'meaningful' activity [viii]– suggesting that the social value placed on having children hasn't decreased while its perceived sense of illusiveness shows an increase. Having children appears to be a luxury people do not perceive they have the time, and often money, to afford. As mothers, due to this epoch of 'professionalised parenting' where we attempt to elevate standards and outcomes of mothering, we are too busy with motherhood to actually benefit from mothering – a kind of sentiment akin to wanting to stop parenting your children so you are able to just enjoy them. Having children becomes a strange but onerous privilege which leads to the many dichotomies that constitute present day parenting.

Despite this, society depends on mothering specifically – and parenting more generally – in a way that it doesn't any other area of human skill or expertise. For this reason, and many more, it is a passionately contested subject we all feel we have a claim to. It's the beginning of the civic individual, society, the nation. The often unseen, rarely heard labour force keeping the country ticking over are mums in their droves. It is simultaneously the everyday and the revolutionary. The most overlooked and the most catered to, the greatest asset to the economy and the greatest drain on it, the most neglected faction of society and the most spoilt – depending on how you choose to look at it.

Positions on motherhood are rhetorical shorthands for a range of political and economic outlooks and so, very often, people with very little understanding of it are more invested and vocal than they have the license to be. It serves as an ideological plinth for both men and women when it comes to debate, a performative tool used in self-congratulatory ways to denote the speaker's position on a whole range of issues.

Part of the knee-jerk, emotive responses to the topic lies in the way motherhood tightropes between the personal and political in such an acute way. Our very nascent beings are shaped by these women who raise us; our basic notion of love, relationality and self are developed through this one relationship. We come to this hive of debate, opinion and discourse with such intimate and personal baggage, that it is hard to make logical sense of it. Society at large recognises the existential value of motherhood also – so socially we approach it with a kind of subconscious disquiet concerning humanity's very survival, and with all the hope and dismay concerning what shape that may take. This is often why these debates are easily – and laughably – racialised, because they adopt the civilisational angst that comes with it too. Discourse around motherhood also becomes more extreme at the political fringes of society, which itself is telling of the kind of tin-foil hat-ism it evokes.

Men and women often weaponise motherhood either for or against their ideals of femininity and each other. This is because being a mum is *falsely* the litmus for the highly contested idea of 'womanhood', and so in keeping with that disputed notion – motherhood is used to both eulogise women and tear them down. The fable of motherhood is so precious in public imagination that we can simply never, as living, breathing women ourselves, live up to its image; to be as blemish free and perfect as the seamless, porcelain concept of 'mum' and all that she means to all of us individually and collectively.

This is why all our tributes to motherhood are elegiac – fitting in with the very temporally contested notion of mothering discussed in the previous chapter – socially we almost always idealise motherhood in *past* tense. Ironically, this is despite the fact that history always forgets the mother. We admonish present day embodiments of motherhood, and laud those historic, more pure and virtuous ones, despite defanging them of any real world impact. Culturally, we do not afford mums the physical and intellectual grace in the present – because that requires more physical and intellectual work on our part; we do not want to disburden them from the labours of motherhood, nor do we want to admit that this burden exists. Motherhood itself must always be a romanticised realm, and anything that distracts from this idealism we create interferes with this love story we sell to ourselves concerning the purest sentiment we can imagine. The passive looking back and admiring motherhood from the buffered distance of time, means we can ignore how rough it is around the edges, how viscerally and cerebrally onerous it is. We can leave the impression of motherhood unimpeached in our individual and collective consciousness so that we may benefit from it in present tense.

As the internet protrudes evermore into our private lives, this tension is heightened for mums who must always be the polished impression of everyone's dream mother; we must be everything to everyone without exception. It's another example of how, by certain social standards, we simply cannot win. Every domain of discourse – be it tabloid news media comment sections, long-read articles, romcoms, and mum blogs themselves – almost the entire infosphere, contributes to an idealised version of motherhood that no one quite recognises but which we all play along with to some extent. An ideation that we as individual women have to carry the burden of – with all the complexity of emotions, and the sense of entitlement, that others bring to the debate.

Most depressingly, these faux-ideals are often wielded by women, against women, to either reduce someone's worth or condescendingly attribute more. You are either betraying women for not setting your sights high enough outside of mothering, or compromising on your femininity for doing too much outside of it. Practically speaking, as mothering is perceived as one of the most quotidian, banal and everyday tasks, it invites the kind of dismissive and derisive responses from those that paradoxically feel they are either above, or not enough to fill the proverbial boots of mothering. You are either derided for being 'just' a mum, or nobody can believe how noble you are for being content with being 'just' a mum, stuck in a perpetual cycle of being too much or not enough and often both at the same time. Women are being bombarded with messages saying motherhood is simultaneously everything and nothing.

And so while we all sit in the violent sways of the pendulum of public opinion which tells us being a mother is what it means to be a woman, and choosing motherhood is a betrayal to true womanhood; while we overcome the motion sickness in the ground shift of conversation which frames it as the single most important thing we can do, and a shackle we need to free ourselves from, we lose focus of a role that is undoubtedly integral to every single one of us individually and the single most important labour force globally.

This dichotomous shaping and response to mothering is strangely telling. In a world structured in binaries, nothing comes close to the concept of mother, it has no equal or counterpart. Motherhood is the kind of role and concept that language and discourse will never quite be able to fully entrap. While economists around the world will tell you what mothers are worth to the economy, while we will be told, rightly, that the domestic and emotional labour can and should be remunerated, the fact remains that the role and impact of motherhood is simply unquantifiable. The fuel that motivates women to give up huge quantities of their emotional and physical existence, simply cannot be framed in labour, economic or transactional terms. It exists in the historically derided domain of immaterial, intuitive, emotional and unempirical. It frustrates those scientists among us who want an easy, definable answer to everything.

Muslim mothers will be subject to additional social expectations – often coloured by their racial and ethnic backgrounds – but also through their identity as Muslims specifically, tethered to the very specific and highly lauded positioning motherhood carries in our faith. While this fact – that as mothers Allāh grants us distinction through His Mercy – is best used as a personal resource for us to draw upon in those many instances that we need them as caretakers of other human souls, it is often used socially to punish us for falling short of these unrealistic and imaginary ideals.

And the equally binary world of the internet which has admittedly done so much for our understanding and implementation of motherhood, often adds further polemics to this issue.

Socially Not-working

It is also worth pointing out here the inherent contradictions of social media. A network designed to bring us closer together, but which creates a strange and voyeuristic proximity, sometimes entirely devoid of what makes human interactions meaningful. As individuals plugging our being, lives and feelings into a system which, by the inevitable consequence of its design, denaturalises our social interactions, this can impact how we treat both ourselves and others. Social media creates a physical barrier between our intimate thoughts and emotions and their very public expression, in the shape of the send button, forcing the critical eye of self-surveillance onto all of our actions. The very public and expressive nature of these platforms means the kind of self-consciousness of a surveyor is forced upon and internalised by most users of social media, consequently, shrouding all of our online interactions in the clinical light of self-awareness, and creating a kind of social mime, a pretension, and a forced persona. In this way it is the antithesis of motherhood, which comes with all its realness, physicality and sobering qualities.

Social media will have you carefully orchestrating a candid, spontaneous moment of your children in beige to juxtapose the blue, seemingly off-the-cuff moment in your feed, three squares down. Typing a deliberately worded, multiply edited caption that's intended to appear nonchalant and aloof. Creating multiple snapshots to add to the carefully curated and heavily edited image you are constructing of your real, everyday life. Emitted out into the chaos and pollution of a social network of over a billion users, under the guise of wanting to create intimate, human connections. All to paint a picture of a fulfilling and whole life which exists outside of the 1080 x 1080 pixel restrictions, and which has you refreshing your feed every five minutes to monitor engagements in 138 x 67 millimeter screens. The dopamine hit that will only ever have us chasing the next high of social approval by likes, retweets, comments and emojis, altering our sense of value and inexorably consuming everyday life.

The aim of many of these platforms – including Instagram and Facebook – is to exploit a vulnerability in human psychology through this 'social-validation feedback loop' as insiders in the tech industry candidly admit.[ix] The prestige that we are hardwired to seek as humans can now be quantified through the immediacy of clicks. This exploitation of what's vulnerable in us reverberates through the entire ecosystem of the online world – not just the infrastructure of design, but the DNA of its content too. Almost every professional content maker is attempting to do this in some respect – create that sweet spot of content that will have us incessantly coming back for more, a stake in one of the biggest industries of our time – the attention economy.

The rise of digital media platforms such as TikTok, combined with smartphones, facilitates the dopamine reward for consuming content with more immediacy, and in a more piecemeal, instant manner. This is exacerbated by these platforms increasingly using scrolling and reeling interfaces where these stimuli optimise what cultural commentators call the 'dopamine doom loop', creating zombie-like, compulsive habits of scrolling and swiping to keep our brains stimulated.[x] The internet has changed both the way we interact with each other and our recreational habits irreparably, and beyond recognition.

At the current pace of innovation in tech and media, this is only developing at break-neck speed. Take the debate during the pre-internet age, regarding high-brow and thought provoking variations of art versus lowly, trash-like entertainment – people often asked whether society was on a downward spiral because rather than, for example, celebrating lofty works of art, we were immersed in serialised TV – effectively devolving from *Faust* to *Friends*. Arguably, our collective attention spans have shrunk even further, as is evident in the insatiable online appetite for short-form video content – often second-long reels – with views in their millions.[xi] The quality and frequency of our social interactions mirror this flattening and accelerating trend – we are better connected, but arguably more lonelier and less meaningfully engaged with each other than ever. Collectively, we have descended from using the medium of theatre, the written word, the celluloid film, and currently digitally hosted, seconds long soundtracked clips to attempt to tell our stories and, now, to make human connections . We are a culture hooked on sheer distraction rather than what we previously looked down upon as entertainment and social engagement, amidst a technological backdrop of infinite, limitless, never ending content for us to doomscroll our way through, in the futile search for meaning, for perpetuity. What this does to us individually is breed an almost constant sense of restlessness, discontentment, unease and headiness. How eerily similar is this to the state of intoxication we are explicitly warned against in the *Quran*, which similarly inhibits our ability to understand and enact our faith in full consciousness? Our phones present eternal opportunities to be anywhere but here; a constant prospect of something else with more potential than the here and now. Motherhood, with its inevitable focus on that here and now outside the screen, is an inconvenient obstacle in Silicon Valley's planned trajectory towards endless profit – it is the ultimate, stubborn human connection in its path.

Communicating, as we increasingly are, through public facing social media platforms means the very purpose of our communication becomes more complex in itself. The gamification of social interaction has us vying for its flattened metrics; our expressive capacity, and therefore our ability to relate to other humans, is reduced to mere buttons on a screen. It is a system designed for audience capture by behemoth tech companies, who hire leading experts in behaviour and psychology, just so they're able to see us as impersonal dots on a graph mapping their own profit.[xii] Because of the way we see ourselves in this equation, social media encourages us to create brands of our own personhood, and market ourselves into product. It breeds a social impulse to turn ourselves into content itself; something easier to visually and culturally consume. We begin to plot ourselves against the topography of commodity. It is the ultimate end to late-stage capitalism, where we become part of that information processing system which is used to asses, market and sell more. We become an active proponent in the machine of capital. By extension, our relationships – with ourselves and others – forms the basis of a new exchange in which communication is a means for commodification.

This content obsessed world means we are offering up our whole lives, and consuming others', as entertainment and distraction amongst voyeuristic and highly critical audiences we perform to and assimilate within; an army of faceless, formless consumers. We have the potential to become both perpetrators and victims of this braying ritual. Quite like the solitary and senseless ramblings of a madman – we are forever interacting with perceived and imaginary spectators, and lengthening and truncating ourselves on that basis, while insisting others do the same.

How we feel, perceive and therefore market ourselves, is shaped by the internet tribes that dominate – for mothers, it may be the crunchy mother, almond mother, or any number of variations of 'mumfluencers' that promote a constructed, and proselytised, way of parenting – and this, of course, shaped by indicators set by tech giants who host our social fetishisation. Our identities are socially constructed by the media we encounter, and the subcultures of today are the new demographics, designed entirely to make us more marketable – these digital tribes represent aspirational and attitudinal markers we adorn our lifestyles with, and we are primarily consumers, not mothers, in this new exchange. Issues as every day to motherhood and therefore which conversely, inevitably, become ideological – such as how long to breastfeed, to vax or not to vax, and what age to let our older children have access to phones and media – are subject to the internal politics of the screen, and mothers are inclined to make decisions on whether or not to engage in baby-led weaning, for example, based on collective identities and group think rooted in commercialism. In this internet hurtled trajectory towards making ourselves more consumable, we have come to brand, and therefore reduce, all of these facets of our thinking and being. We become mere logos, competing for advertising space, and kudos, on this digital terrain. The internet feeds this moral laziness and social neediness in us; it is that black mirror that obscures the reflection we see of ourselves.

As such, despite the wealth of information now at our fingertips, we are stylising and commodifying parenting – one of the realest and most personal endeavours we can embark upon – through the medium of the internet which demands, really, our most surface-level self. In many ways, the essence of motherhood desists the screen because it is too true a substance for its shallow capacity, and this is something we must bear in mind when we give or take to the lore of parenting online. Our children exist outside the vortex of the internet – their whole, nuanced self, and all the quirks they embody, will not always follow the formulas we find through this labyrinth. In the same way, we are seeking our very real need for support and companionship in our often solitary capacity as mothers through a network which will always reduce us to our most commodified selves, a reality we must also be cognisant of when we turn to these cold glass walls for social fulfilment. And as consumers of this media, we are becoming increasingly invested in these digital constructs of parenting, and the faces that promote them.

This has a natural domino effect on our endeavours to learn, grow and socially connect as parents. Due to the pressure for content makers to attention-farm, the click-bait, inane fodder we often get as a result is not always useful or meaningful. Collectively, there appears to be a trajectory of consuming mum content for shallow personal-brand affirmation or mere diversion alone. Because we have created trends of parenting that are often needlessly tribalistic and therefore reduce mothering to an arbritrary set of stylised rules, our digital consumption as mothers is not always productive. Often, it very much fits into the bracket of distraction and an unproductive form of escapism; in how it feeds our ego, clouds our thinking, encourages a focus on outward expression, rather than internal reflection, but also particularly as our mothering is dependent on personal relationships with our children, which take time, effort, and mental space to foster.

For Muslim mothers for whom motherhood is now in danger of falling into distraction, entertainment and performance, the very standards which we internalise and parent by are impacted. As the relationship between the private and public bends and warps, so do our very notions of what it means to mother. We are publicly expressing to the world the kind of mother we are, often according to a set of rules or conventions predetermined by the algorithms of the online world, and we are judging other mothers by this same standard. This impacts on our intimate impressions of ourselves as Mums, with an inexhaustible capacity for self-recrimination. Amongst all of this, there are, of course, a number of high profile Muslim mothers online who are producing meaningful content that is directional, purposeful, and therefore popular amongst Muslim mums, and this is amongst some of the many benefits we do inevitably get from these human centred systems – despite the profit inclinations that belie them.

Despite this, there is a growing body of evidence which demonstrates what the pattern of compulsive consumption, and the nature of what we consume on the information highway, is damaging to young digital natives' mental wellbeing.[xiii] Less is said about how much this impacts us as mothers specifically; how parenting in a world saturated with social media poses a threat to agency, sincerity, and meaningful development and growth. Our time, and attention, is the internet's most precious commodity. Our phones, and the social media we have access to via them, are designed purely to keep our minds engaged, and therefore too occupied to invest in relationships that sit outside of the screen. While we might be conscious of our children's access to digital devices, we are less vigilant of the idea that internet trends equally have the potential to warp our own sense of maternal perception. We are, often wilfully, ignorant to how opening ourselves up to a world of opine, judgement and criticism can arrest our growth and hold our happiness, as mothers, hostage.

Coupled, of course, with the many ways that the inevitable act of comparing yourself to others in this shiny utopia of the screen impacts us, and we are effectively setting ourselves up to fail in many ways.

Mirror, mirror, on the wall...

The debate concerning the internet's capacity to create narrow, punishing norms and ideals is well known and understood, and the wrongs of this well documented. What is less explored, but more insidious, is what the counter narrative to promote realistic standards on the internet also reveals about and reinforces in us, and what that says about how we use the internet, a tool which has irremediably changed our social interactions. Because social media, in its very essence, repels the 'real' – it is designed entirely to help us escape it. It is a social contract we've all signed to leave our actual, unfiltered selves at the virtual door. Reality is too ugly for a world that we have consciously shaped through our collective efforts of delusion. We are, like irrepressible herds, drawn in our trance to elements of this "real" – the image outside the digital cave – and that's why certain tweets or memes resonate with us, because they remind us of the sunlight beyond the blinds we draw to shade it, about something within us that is actual and unmediated. If we believe culture has subsumed us entirely and there are no natural reflexes or instincts untouched by those social forces, then the digital age has intensified that process and by consequence our own latent thirst for authenticity in an increasingly fake world. Despite this unspoken rule to bar what's real and tangible from our online world, most of us are familiar with the conversations, internet movements and media campaigns to promote realistic standards on the internet; to show non-airbrushed, unstaged, candid insights into people's lives, ostensibly so that we all have a healthier self-image. And some of these are, of course, warranted, needed and justified, as we have explored through the ideation of motherhood. This increasingly normative attitude of forcing realism on the simulation of the online realm can also, however, lead to a fixation on other people's weaknesses and a complacency when it comes to our own. A trait that has always existed in us as social animals, but which our new glossy toy that is the internet amplifies in many ways.

There is this newly emergent refrain that we repeat to ourselves as we scroll through the endless world of dopamine-trapped content, which summarises so perfectly all that is wrong with how we interact with these recreational tools that have come to dwarf and redefine our own material lives. A supposedly reassuring but discordant chant, a scurrilous taunt at content makers, by us as fellow content makers, that's picking up momentum and volume. It kicks in once that creeping, fearful emotion swells up gradually inside us; when we are confronted with the perfect table setting, the neatly turned out, smiling children, and the ideal looking Mum to frame it.

Bet she doesn't look like that in real life.

It's just a filter.

No one's house is that clean.

She's probably maxed out four credit cards.

They're definitely arguing all the time.

And with that soothing, dulcet chime now playing in your heads, a palpable sense of relief subdues that incipient sense of insecurity – we move onto the next post and the next chorus of self-placating put downs: drag, release, refresh.

What underpins our own need to ask others to offer their more 'real' self to the world, when we understand and participate in a system that will always present a mediated version of ourselves to it?

The filters we employ when we put our lives out on display in the court of public opinion, literal or metaphorical, have set a dangerous precedent of unattainable standards and unrealistic expectations – the opinion piece tells. *And that's why we must tear this illusion down, bit by bit. Post by post and poster by poster*, is how we rationalise it.

While we all want to present the best side of ourselves on social media, there are elements of ourselves that begrudge others doing the same. Undoubtedly there is something noble in the movement to create more realistic standards on social media – but this is often done disingenuously because we feel *we* are owed a stake in public adoration and praise. The dormant instinct in us to drag others down to make ourselves feel better is aroused when we are so subject to motherhood-as-mime in a globalised age. With a social network that connects us to millions, rather than tens, of other mothers, our perception of ourselves is both shrunk and constricted, and inflated and decontextualised in ways that is not always productive, and that can lead to a lack of perspective and growth.

We all know that social media exists to help us to escape reality, and yet we're all ostensibly screaming for it to be more 'real'; and what we often mean by this reality we seek, is a Sims-like incubator where we feel most comfortable, unperturbed in the brand we've created for ourselves. We all seek out validation through these apps, yet we decry the influence of those most validated. Should we be trying to create more realistic standards in beauty, living and relationships or should we be trying to create more healthy and realistic standards in our appetite for public applaud? And is it not an important part of our development as mothers to recognise plurality, both when we are understanding other people's reality, and in how we recognise our own?

And these feelings are all the more complex because of the social pressures of being a mum. Personally, we feel we have something to prove as society's perception of us as mothers makes up our own most intimate sense of self-worth. When beauty ceases to be the main barometer of womanhood, "motherhood", as it's socially constructed as a standard, can take over and be equally hostile and unproductive grounds for women. And because the weight of the world is brought onto the doorstep of mothering, we are inheriting everyone else's baggage. The smog of content that exists defining, redefining, shaping, reshaping, judging and condemning mothers is suffocating. The steely gaze of motherhood becomes equally punishing and obscures our sense of growth.

This sentiment which underlies what might be better described as relationships-as-consumption, really just epitomises our latent need to want to be better, while affording others less. To apply the filter to our own world, while looking into others' without that same sense of grace and generosity. Ironically, it is symptomatic of a therapy culture gone mainstream, a double-speak which always puts the onus on others for your own sense of growth, development, agency and fault. Allāh asks us to look at those 'below' us to engender the necessary gratitude for our blessings, and yet we seek that sense of social comparison to generate a better self and public image, and create a grandiose version of ourselves, rather than to contextualise ourselves in necessary ways. It exposes an insecurity and fatalism in us, that an all-or-nothing culture of mothering has created, put on steroids through the filtered white-light projected from the internet. We cannot afford to acknowledge personal flaw when we are committed to such public perceptions of ourselves. Error or weakness presents an end to the shiny, marketable end-products, we present ourselves as, rather than a means for learning and self-growth. And that is because the internet will almost always have us smoothing over the public cracks, at the expense of our internal reserves and strength.

There are other ways social media has exacerbated weaknesses in our need for social value and approval. These networks effectively mean we can never experience the natural life cycle of female friendships, the spontaneity and organic movement of people in and out of our lives – both the balance and sweet subtleties inherent in that social pattern, and also what it teaches us about impermanence, temperance and valuing others' presence. We are bound, through these digital chains, to each other, and are constantly visibly, accessible – and in some ways socially accountable – to anyone we've ever been in any proximity with; be it the girl we went to secondary school with, or the office manager at our last job. Sometimes this desire to remain vigilant of, and even visible to, other women on the peripheries of our existence can breed unhealthy habits. We can, if we are not careful, begin to assess other women almost as threat levels – we may want to, or be encouraged to by the function of social media design, use other women's perceived worth to validate our own. Weigh them up on the scale between ordinary and remarkable, specifically so we can measure ourselves by that same social ranking. This interest can of course come from a healthy and productive place, but it can almost just as likely come from a sense of perverse intrigue that privileges superficial notions of the self.

Memeification and a new social refrain

Because of this focus on the self as a highly visible brand, and our reduced relationality to others, social media has the potential to nurture an obsessive main-character syndrome. Think of how the language developed within the digital domain fixates on the primacy of self – OOTD, POV, NPC[10] and the more explicit 'main character energy'– the internet is imbuing us with the linguistic tools to create an overblown sense of our own subject, employing the global reach we have access to via its network as a means for self-promotion. This hyperbolic and self-centring internet refrain targets, and holds a specific kind of weight with, women because we deem it as an affront to, and kicking back of, the centuries-long worth of subjugation we've endured. For so long a specific kind of sacrifice was expected of women because of falsified ideals concerning femininity,

---

[10] Outfit of the day, point of view, non-player character

with Muslim women bearing the brunt of this, and Muslim mums in particular expected to reduce the social and political space they inhabit almost entirely. While it remains that we still need to rediscover and reassert our worth within our social settings, superficial and counterproductive approaches to this which often go against the grain of our faith, are merely palliative, they give us the illusion of movement and progress when in reality they are smokescreens for true advancement. Often softer forms of activism in the digital domain – which include a certain kind of bravado – are just useful distractions from the real world through which we gain our sense of self-confidence and rights. This phenomenon creates an internet driven solipsism and a kind of self-centring which we qualify through the style of activism – ultimately it conflates historical, structural issues with personal ones, and privileges ourselves, falsely, as the site for these solutions. It is a trend which inflates our own fragile opinion of ourself, making us more prone to self-indulgence and self-criticism in equal measure. Both these qualities arrest maternal progress in their extremes – we are either fawning over ourselves too much to cultivate the kind of sincerity integral to parenting, or self-reproaching ourselves into inertia. The stupefying nature of social media, if we are not careful, can extend to our moral inclinations too.

The human need to want to be valid, seen, recognised is not something we are encouraged to interrogate or temper when we all have the means of self-publicisation. As we are so invested in our own personal brand, and the narrative-arc we've created for ourselves, any misgiving presents a hole in this sense of self-perception we've created for ourselves and our sense of self-esteem by which it hangs. A fear of being ousted or relegated by the global digital tribe consequently governs so much of what we do, 'cancel culture' has entered our intimate thought space.

And this is without delving into what social media speak cultivates in us – a kind of socially-approved 'meanness', that we mistake for authenticity which has such currency in the simulation of the online world. In reality this distinctly digital brand of authenticity is bred from an instinct to appear aloof and detached, which is embedded in its very parlance of 'brat summers' and the like. This idea that we must promote an exaggerated sense of self-confidence in ourselves, while being highly, openly, and vocally critical of others is part of the DNA of internet culture. It is such a persuasive and irresistible diction, that it is almost impossible to engage in internet culture without this recalcitrant, reproachful and retorting refrain.

The architectural features of the internet themselves hint at the potential dangers of the kind of intensified and expanded peer pressure we experience through social media use – the very memefication of communication itself, which is heralded as a social emollient, is not always the positive and joyous thing it's made out to be. The Kamala Harris 2024 presidency campaign was notoriously steered by a digitally savvy meme intelligence –itself symbolic, given her resistance to creating any kind of meaningful change in foreign policy. How we, as a community of users, sometimes engage in the social language of the internet, how we perceive and employ memes is also telling. The clips, extracts and distillations of cultural events that become canonised in our collective dictionary of memes carry on in that same spirit that generated them; they are moments of common expression – be it disgust, humour, dismay or mockery – crystalised in popular memory. They immortalise these feelings and sentiments and cement them in our cultural muscle memory. The memes of today become our shared language and values of tomorrow.

What's worrying about this is that these moments which are ironically built upon shared sentiment are often exclusionary; in how they deride and sneer at any given person, symbol or culture. They epitomise the contradictory nature of ourselves as social animals, and our use of the internet in this kingdom – in that our feelings of togetherness and solidarity are often built upon the barring of others. Our proclamations of other people's or group's moral or social inferiority come from a paradoxical assertion of our apparent superiority. It seems that the only way to create cultural unity is by manufacturing pockets of disunity. Despite, and perhaps because of, this relatively 'socially conscious' epoch of youth culture, where we are arguably most careful about a certain kind of moral offence centred on identity politics, we are unable to resist a good ganging-up and cussing down of someone for some innocuous act, and the feelings of supremacy it gives rise to.

Very often, despite the progressive values we wear so proudly, the things we collectively and unquestioningly deride, mock, or laugh at serve as proxies for marginalised identities such as working class or racialised cultures – see the plethora of TikToks mocking white working-class 'Fiat 500' culture and denigrating these aesthetics and lifestyle choices. Because we forget how ingrained we all are in a capitalist system which depends upon an underclass, and how this plays out along the lines of race and gender in common culture (extending even into intracommunity politics of American Muslims versus British Muslims, or even more locally, London Muslims versus Bradford Muslims...). Indeed, we can look at these cultural moments, the memes, internet discourse and the sentiment that they've spurned in the social laboratory of the internet, and learn a lot about what we try to suppress about us as a culture.

Many will point out the trend amongst Millennial and Gen Z audiences of assigning an ethical value to any given trend they may be drawn to or repulsed by. This is because we have become conditioned to see our likes and dislikes as a sign of our morality, rather than superficial preferences; denoting a constant need to feed our sense of superiority. Less, however, is written about how the inverse is true – how we ignore moral considerations when it comes specifically to our instincts for condescension and snobbery. We may want to focus on our capacity to be principled when it creates a positive self-image, but we are less likely to hold a mirror up to our darker, more insidious tendencies, or to probe into our less desirable sides.

Mothering in the many and everyday

The way many of us are tempted to use the internet, to stoke our ego and assuage our insecurities, runs contrary to how Islam dictates that we be socialised. Very often we use it to exceptionalise the unexceptional; to platform ourselves as protagonists in a world created by us for our own glory. Islam depends on an uncompromisingly dichotomous notion of Creator and man; this is evident in our most prolific act of worship, *sujūd* [11]; when we lay our head to the ground, the lower-most point, we utter his name, and glorify Him in His capacity of *Al-Ala* the Most High. We acknowledge through this instinctual act, the relative position of mankind and our Creator, one that we all unquestioningly submit to and which is encoded in our very existence. Our Lord is One and we are many. Allāh has granted us blessings in that notion of many – we are collectively, in our dependent sense of self, worthy. This doesn't mean we aren't naturally worthy individually, or that we lack intrinsic value, but that that value is positional; we are valuable as *insān*, as Allāh created us, and in our context within fellow creation. Our honouring ourselves is dependent on the recognition that we must honour others

---
[11] Prostration

by that same token too. We must, of course, love for our brothers what we love for ourselves. The nuances of this are beautiful and enriching to the mind and soul. They are entirely necessary for us as individuals and parents. And while consumer driven capitalist culture has us framing our value in individualism and being uniquely worthy, we become blind to the collective element of our existence that actually grants us more dignity and honour. We also become drawn into a system which privileges one form of success, from being seen and validated at the expense of others, and which therefore creates just enough room for women to fight for scraps, rather than support each other and hold each other up.

A more pluralistic understanding of maternal success, based on a social contract which is rooted in Islamic objectives, in which we honour one another and recognise the blessings Allāh has given us all in our various situations, gives us the agency and ability to succeed and nurture each other as we do so. Contentment comes from understanding that your situation is unique and different, part of the journey Allāh has blessed us with, and our collective goal is that effort, seeking and endeavour to be better believers, and aid others to do the same, with our blessings.

The *rizq*[12] Allāh grants us through our social, emotional, personal and economic wealth, which is written for us.

The human desire to exceptionalise oneself is embedded in the very structures of our existence and in what we embellish our culture in. The whole notion of classism and fashion rests upon this premise of hierarchy that we have an innate capacity to feed into. Is it any wonder the internet has fed the beast of our ego, and created an influx of ways to gauge and quantify ourselves with and against.

If, personally, in how we perceive and project ourselves to the world, our social media use, and the footprint it leaves behind, we aim to create this forged sense of 'natural' from the unnatural, and want to exceptionalise the unexceptional, then we are further away from the reality of Islam which is situated in the everyday. The routine moments that make up our existence and the quotidian actions that pepper them, the deeds we amass; that very dimension in which happiness has its throne also, and where contentment perches – the momentary existence that we inhabit. The internet, both in how we use it as mindless distraction, an alternative universe,

---

[12] Provision, sustenance or a gift

and as a literal platform to the world for our online persona and life, creates an appetite for short, sharp highs that we suspend our sense of worth and self-perception from. And when it's the inebriating influence of this internet that we use as a crutch to help us to get through a day of reality and comparative, perceived banality, the real world pales in comparison to what our hand held, pleasure-rewarding machine can offer. And this instant-gratification-seeking-behaviour that the internet and social media are engineered to bring out in us, extends to our approach to faith. Very often we are drawn to *da'ees*[13] that provide us with sound bites that deliver that immediacy – rapid bursts of *imaan*, and this is at expense of the enduring knowledge and reality that paint the intricacies and subtleties of being Muslim. The everyday, every-minute, Islam that embellishes our lives with things that make it directional, purposeful, in submission and obedience to Him. It's the reassurance that we carry that the wider picture – including the smaller difficulties and triteness that constitute it – is part of something meaningful that we are invested in and that we know is ultimately more than what we might immediately perceive. *Imaan* also exists

---

[13] Caller to Islam

in the difficult, in having *sabr*,[14] getting through the eleventh hour of parenting with playdough in your hair, biting your tongue – it's not just the superficially constructed high. It is also where we will find the kind of quiet peace and cognisance that acts as a balm to the soul, and the slow release caffeine necessary for our day.

Islam gives us so much beauty in the everyday, and the temperance in seeking more, which we often become disenchanted with and removed from due to the constant stimulation of the online world, and our dopamine-wired existence. There is meaning and enrichment in the detail, and dare I say it, humility in the slog. The balance of being main, side, and background character, of understanding the ecosystem of our society without privileging yourself as the individual solely and persistently. This is especially important as we mother, because every impulse will be telling you to exceptionalise your child, when it is them being conscious of their place and context in the world that will grant them the qualities of a believer, God willing.

The online world, which interlaces the public and private spheres, disrupts that very sense of time and being. It distorts our sense of temporality,

---
[14] Patience

and our capacity to exist in, and enjoy the here and now. A here and how which is effectively the soil from which we mother; that creates the subtle hues that make parenting enjoyable and meaningful – that luxury we spoke of earlier, and often the persistent ingredient for maternal happiness. Frequently, as mothers, with mental load, we seek some much contested time and space for ourselves – digital spaces can certainly help to enhance that time if used correctly, but it can also corrupt it too. Time itself is experiential, it is a *rizq* that comes directly from Allāh, and we are abundant and rich in it when we direct it towards Him.

Motherhood is tempered by the bittersweet after taste of impermanence – the relative hardship we face, but also the happiness and joy our growing children bestow upon us is brief and transitory. And even this is something we experience in a disjointed way – our children do not inhabit the same time zone as us. Their nascent experiences are new and fresh, and therefore long and drawn out, while ours are rapid and forgettable from the constant weathering of life. The screens we willingly appoint as crutches often diminish these fleeting and fragile moments that we will never be able to recoup. From those moments that will become their core memories and that we are so blessed with in that moment, once ours have hardened and crystalised.

Motherhood as the opposite of our social-media world

In a 280 character, external-facing, gratifying, online world, which privileges neat, measurable and definable reposts, follows and shares, and the immediacy of the satisfaction it brings, motherhood sits in defiant juxtaposition as an ever-changing series of goal posts, as an often unseen, unquantifiable role that is constant, enduring, twisting and turning. There is no running counter of likes, there isn't always the fire emoji wielding comment to give you that external boost. And in acknowledging the quaintness of that, there is benefit. It's doing the work that only Allāh sees and only He rewards. In situating your effort in the silence of Allāh's sight alone, in the blessing of having your deeds visible only to Him. The quiet space where barakah is replete and where *imaan* is nurtured and grows. Much of motherhood exists in this invisible-to-the-human-eye and unquantifiable dimension of *barakat*, not in the measure of economics or social media metrics.

The fact is motherhood is difficult, often a little dull and monotonous, but nothing good comes easy, and we are never meaningfully stretched, pushed and bolstered without a level of strife. Discomfort, and in some instances boredom, is absolutely necessary for growth as we do and will teach our children time and time again. And the benefits of motherhood are amongst the best kind for personal and spiritual growth. Your sense of achievement will never quite be satiated; there is always that extra thing to work on, that habit to help overcome, that milestone that is further down the road of development. It creates a sense of temperance and endurance that will motivate you to keep climbing, force you to regroup, collect yourself in the moment and take stock of the long term.

The TikTok-ification of everyday life where everything is outward performance baits us into wanting to create a narrative arc for public consumption. Ultimately, the narrative pattern that we are creating through our social media presence, and our offline acts that prop it up, is meaningless – as fleeting as the light and colour of the many pixels that forge this vision. It is distraction, screen-fodder, another opportunity for others to judgementally swipe. Recognising that we are in control of our real narrative arc, and this is only visible to, and judgement and praise from it lies only with Allāh, helps us to wean ourselves off the treadmill of constant seeking of public approval and adoration. The respite Allāh gives us in the private, the solace He bestows in introspection, is worth rediscovering. We say it countless times every day, but to embody the notion that all praise belongs to and comes from Him is where our sense of reality and grounding comes from. To dislocate our sense of achievement and success from the ostentation of the screen and the flattering of our own person, and resituate it in the context of the abilities Allāh has endowed us with, and the social structures that may have supported it. In doing this, you acknowledge you are exceptional because Allāh has granted you that within the myriad of blessings we are all endowed with, always. The extended beauty of this, of course, is the fact that we refrain from the short lived raptures of self-adoration and praise, and the inevitable come down and deflation we experience when we attach our sense of self-worth to material objects and achievements, off-screen and on.

Imaan is undoubtedly the most precious element of our being – an entirely uncommodifiable, invisible-to-the-human-eye trait, and one that requires true cultivation, and for which we can take some credit for, as it is borne of the choices Allāh has blessed us with. And really, it is all we have. It is the only thing that remains with us in a transient and increasingly cruel world. It is what defines us in material and immaterial plains, and it is the only quality worth nurturing. How we nurture this *imaan* or faith, is completely devoid of the public, watchful nature of the internet, in fact it could not be more antithetical to it. It is the realest endeavour we will ever embark upon and we will rarely find it reflected in or encouraged by the acts of cultural consumption we often engage in, it requires a self-reckoning that some corners of the internet work to stifle entirely. The kernel of *imaan* comes from the recognition that we can fool others, those – real or imagined – that we create social media posts for, for example. But we cannot fool ourselves or Allāh; irrespective of our digital narratives, we are contributing to a real narrative – one intertwined with our inner most thoughts and motivations – and from that private space our relationship with Allāh exists. The relationship we have with Allāh, which is so intimately tied to our sense of self-honesty, is one that desists from all these internet-heady delusions. It requires introspection, honesty and integrity.

And in saying all of this, I am not promoting an appetite for punishment. This is not the oft-told story about women having to endure pain, sacrifice or misery as part of their biological, and what's often construed as 'religious', destiny, rather it is reimagining what true happiness and contentment looks like, and what shape that truly takes in our life. Motherhood is an awesome and sublime experience. And we glean so much from it. But the body of work that sits below the tip of that beautiful iceberg is often what is most vilified and feared by women in equal measure. And it's also what creates the strength, endurance and weight to hold the crown of it atop. It is without doubt the discomfort that guarantees exponential personal and spiritual growth. So, this is the tale of us as believers, and reevaluating what is advantageous to us in that non-gendered capacity of *mu'min*[15] alone. And it encompasses our role as mothers, which is anchored in our very being. This is the unique task Allāh sent to us specifically as women, with all the physical, mental and religious implications it brings to our doorsteps here and the hereafter.

Once we compartmentalise our screens as a mere accessory to meaningful living, rather than the

---

[15] Believer

means through which we live, we start to see how being a mother means that socially you will inhabit more space, and your interests and concerns will mirror that. You will develop a voracious appetite for child development, learning, character development. A desire to learn that is so honestly and wholesomely anchored in a sincerity and want to be and do better. You will start to look at the political machinations behind everyday aspects of being. You will also start to see the world as a canvas for the future – what kind of backdrop should we be wanting for our children and all children like them.

Islamically we have to foster a languid and unending pool of unconditional love for our children, one which nurtures, rewards and prioritises their growth as believers – not that indulges them into inaction and complacency. As well as the physical and emotional demands of motherhood, creating this capacity for an almost-other-worldly kind of love is a constant and active endeavour. Islam tells us to love with limits when it is most difficult to – in how we cosset children, and shape their character and moral capacity for good. And Islam tells us to love without limits when we most want to impose them – in how we offer our duty and care. It's a love that's disciplined, and purified and mediated through our relationship with the Creator. Personally, it is a laboured and sometimes painful effort, but done with the right intentions we are promised rewards from He who is the arbiter of all truth.

If having a child means creating new habit formations, then persist with those that bring us closer to Allāh, rather than those which take us further away. Understanding the internet in its context means recognising that those boundaries by which you self-evaluate should be firmly entrenched in the Quran and Sunnah alone, and that is the constant, disciplining force in our lives; how each of us with our unique personalities come to adopting and enforcing that often involves the part of us that is most damaged by the internet, our intuitive self. And this is particularly the case when you pass on these skills of self-understanding and orienting to your children.

Motherhood is a human endeavour to do the best with what you have, to draw on every resource and economise all your good will, patience and fortitude to best meet the needs of growing, malleable and needy little minds. It is about you and another developing human sharing a life and growing together, with all the complexities and deep joys that brings. It is as much about introspection, emotional intelligence, self-reflection and understanding as it is about following a formula. Very often the online world can stifle these qualities. But motherhood is ultimately the ability to tune your inner self into another cognitive being, being painfully honest about your own human flaws, and receptive and compassionate of theirs. It's that honest and real conversation you can just about bear to have with yourself, extended to another person you have the blessing of guiding through those delicate years of childhood. It exists in that space from which you make dua, from which you understand, so acutely, what really matters and who you really are, stripped of all the worldly paraphernalia.

These intuitive skills will likely already exist in you even when we are used to repressing them for so long. And you will just need to hone and sharpen them to bring out the best in yourself, and the little being whose development you now have the blessing to aid. It is that oft-ignored voice in the back of your head. So much of this work needs to be done using the raw materials of your very self. So much of it is uncomfortable and disciplining. So much of it is resisting the urge to do the easy, 'affirming' thing. And so much of it is in the messy, banal and tedious of the everyday that we spend too much of our time escaping to the internet from.

New frontiers

For many of us in the modern world, who grew up without a sense of community, becoming a mother is the first time we recognise the need, and make effort to seek, that elusive sense of community. That extending of one's interests into another small human, means we begin to value what it means to be human, and an inevitable consequence of that is the tribe, or herd. As relational beings, this sense of community is arguably one of the most important elements of life. How we mediate these relationships, in a digital age where we are seeking those relationships online, and which promotes a kind of detachment, is key. Very often, the online world disorders our sense of what's real – something that will only accelerate as we go teeming towards an AI enhanced world. The screen that borders our digital relationships acts as a kind of nullifying force which disturbs our sense of proportionality and perception of what's right or wrong. It appears to us like a social mirage devoid of real world consequence, when in reality our actions inside and outside of the screen make up the deeds that will sit on our scales on the last day.

This is especially important when we look at how the internet, and the sport of spectating, impresses upon our finer instincts and cognitive habits. If we are constantly fault finding in others to satiate our need for approval – a fire that often rages stronger once you are a mother and subject to a new arena of scrutiny – or as a means to distract from that niggling sense of insecurity, than we must not give that fire the oxygen it needs to grow stronger.

This is why the Sunnah to think more critically of yourselves than others, to tightrope carefully between those twin considerations that define us as believers – fear of and hope in Allāh – and extend a kinder more compassionate narrative to others is such a key human consideration. Creating a happy story – that sense of *hasn al dhan*[16] – which excuses others, is not only part of our faith, and therefore a humane and decent thing to do – it will also help to create a cushioning bubble to better aid your own development. It is acknowledging that the Islamic concept of '*khibr*'[17] which Allāh tells us is nullifying even in atomic weight, includes looking down on others as well as denying His truth. Allāh is Merciful because in what He prescribes us for our difficulties and struggles, He also deposits its cure. The time-honoured tradition – facilitated by consum-

---

[16] Having good thoughts of others
[17] Pride

erist culture – of women looking down upon each other to make themselves feel better is really just the surface wound of the deeper injury that is a culture which makes us feel worthless. When we place the critical eye on others, we create space to become complacent about ourselves. Resisting that descension into needless expressed or unexpressed criticism of others is necessary to foster the space for productivity and growth. It is a sign of our own strength and fortitude.

We know that *shaitan*[18] is man's open enemy and that he is preoccupied with the house of the Muslim because of the very *imaan* we possess. We know that faith can sometimes make us complacent too, a phenomenon akin to what sociologists describe as the licensing effect, which tells us that self-righteous morality is a major cause of immorality. The belief that we are good can create a kind of complacency that makes it easy to fall into bad. Muslims are often cultured into accepting our greater sacrifices in abstaining from those big, lifestyle related harms means we can become lazy when it comes to identifying and harnessing our finer moral characteristics. We feel secure as Muslims in the fact we don't drink alcohol, or eat pork, and from that place of security we might be

---
[18] The devil

more likely to partake in smaller misgivings that aren't as obvious to ourselves or others. Often these smaller imperfections in our moral fibre detract from our shield, not just from further sin, but also our sense of happiness and resilience.

As a civilisation, we are no longer inventing labour-altering machines anymore, and therefore advances in society no longer have such physical implications. The second industrial revolution gave us electricity, motor vehicles and aircraft – advancements that changed the very way we live our lives. The information technology revolution gives us culture-making machines such as phones, TikTok and AI, creating content and culture wars that impact the very way we think, as we will unearth in more depth in the final chapter. Like any tools – they can be used for good; TikTok, which a majority of young people now use as a news source,[xiv] has led to the kind of democratisation of media and knowledge that led to many populist movements against genocide in Gaza, for example (hence the fierce legal battles to have it outlawed in America…) and it is the first platform in which Islam is spoken about without being imbued in shame – a ground-breaking and world-altering thing; we are effectively *'Brother errr'*-ing ourselves into mainstream acceptance. Of course these new digital tools can also be used malignantly, see the uncompromising quest for profit and attempt to monetise our existence that we've discussed. This does not mean, of course, that we engage in a kind of technopessimism and ignore the potential of these new technologies – certainly not in this advent of AI and its ground-breaking possibilities. Social media, digital and technological advancements facilitate our lives, and we can make of them what we want. What it does require, is us interrogating how these tools are used to generate capital and the profiteering models they are moulded into. How this impacts our relationship with ourselves and others. And how we might use new tools to cement age old problems.

Inarguably, the most important relationship in our life is that relationship with Allāh, and we gain so much from using that to mediate all else, rather than falling into the trap of modifying our relationship with Allāh according to our relationship with others. And developing a relationship with Allāh requires knowing Him – in all His Magnitude; Allāh is *al-Ahad*, the Unique, He is Uniquely perfect, He is *al-Barr*, the Source of Goodness, He is characterised by mercy, goodness, and generosity. He is *Al-Ra'oof*, the Compassionate, the One Who consoles broken hearts and He is *Al-Lateef*, the Most

Subtle and Courteous, He understands the most subtle things and takes care of us in ways that we are not even aware of. Everything we have – including the blessing of our children – is from His infinite Mercy, and understanding this gives us the lens through which to see the world through our many blessings. Very often, without this contextual knowledge of ourselves and our Creator, we seek to attach our impaired image of ourselves to something we perceive as greater, to feel part of something bigger; the 'collective fictions' sociologists and anthropologists speak of which we create to give us a sense of meaning and grandiose. Whether it's the social pressures we face before motherhood that we spoke about at the beginning of this chapter, to appear cool and aloof, or being part of a faction of the 'mum' community – be it virtual or material. Some of these collective identities can be empowering but it can also lead us to be partisan in a number of ways, and complacent in others; and these are the pitfalls to avoid in how we parent as social animals. Allāh has given us the greatest collective identity which is rooted in the very pattern of our design; our fitrah. And often, it's those communal fictions, those stories we tell ourself, that can be so dangerously, morally pacifying and ethically nullifying.

CHAPTER 3

THE POLITICAL: THE MUSLIM *(M)*OTHER

> *Verily! This is the true narrative, and La ilaha ill-Allāh. And indeed, Allāh is the All-Mighty, the All-Wise. (Surah Al-Imran 3:62)*

There's something about those crackling, black and white movies and the feeling they elicit. That Sunday afternoon comfort of abandoning yourself in a duvet and an old family favourite, with all of its warm and reassuring familiarity. There is good, there is evil. Good triumphs, credits roll, and we go about our business with that sweet aftertaste of justice and a lingering film score echoing through our day.

Humans are naturally drawn to the sequential pattern of stories. As mothers, we are reminded of this through those persistently trying, book-induced toddler tantrums, and our own childhood memories of torch-light reading and Saturday morning cartoons. As we grow older our affinity for being taken, by hand, through that smooth and predictable journey – cutting into the wilderness of a promising, hopeful beginning, a jungle of a gripping middle, and sailing down through the calm waters of a conclusive and finite end – remains with us. This narrative topography satisfies an innate atavistic appetite – a wish fulfilment to see all the pieces of the puzzle so absolutely in place to reveal a greater image of truth and goodness. It appeals to our most primordial self, and speaks to our desire for a narrative of life, which is itself entirely unpredictable, and which leaves no hint or suggestions to our own inevitable ending. And while that inner thirst for sequence, order and finality is made most obvious to us through cinema, it is a reflection of the models and stories we create in life outside of it.

Though the broader pattern of story, with the reassuring bookmarking of beginning and end, is cathartic to us as social animals, the structural, binary features of 'good' and 'bad' are equally important to our sense of meaning-making. We depend upon this stark, black and white opposition of good to bad, and the certainty and righteousness it brings. We need to see the world defined in these neat, assuring compartments that validate our own moral sense of self. That help us self-aggrandise, and identify with something greater, outside of our individual selves. We determine meaning through these binary structures on both a molecular and broad scale. Psychologically and linguistically we can attribute meaning to 'black' because we know it is the opposite of 'white'. Socially we derive value from the 'good' as the opposite of 'bad'.

These binaries exist within a hierarchical structure that is purposed by our social setting – weak is undesirable and strong is desirable. The predator has value and the victim is devalued. The coloniser ought to be emulated and the colonised degraded and ignored. These symbols form a social contract we are all innately familiar with, which we are born into and which form the confines within which we perceive and live.

Once upon a time...

How society defines and positions the semantic fields that are the building blocks for meaning and value constitutes our world view as social animals. It determines how we, and our children, see and order everything around us. More recent cultural history has seen Hollywood asking us to put our trust in the cowboy, as a beacon of Western progressive liberalism, and to feel disdain towards its perceived opposite, the supposedly savage and obscure 'Red Indian'. This is because as an audience we are supposed to identify with the cowboy, while the indigenous American population is othered into a monster outlier that gives the cowboy purpose and meaning.

While it is external powers in politics, media and culture that mostly shape the stories we live by and which determine our values, we as an audience get something out of the deal too. The dualities they promulgate give the watchful viewer a self-affirmant– that we in our homes, small and vulnerable, are part of a greater, validated identity of 'us'. Outside of the implicit and explicit narratives society operates on, we are insignificant and lacking. It satisfies our constant need for purpose.

These tales which shape our world uphold wider metanarratives; the broader, over-arching stories humanity tells itself, that equally work to confirm our collective, often national, or ethno-national, sense of being. They are the lullabies that soothe, pacify and distract us, en masse, from the complexities of the real world. Think of it like an industrialised version of your own internal running commentary, perennially narrating your life, and through which your sense of self-esteem is based; how we are all constantly writing our own story, defining our world and being so that we feel seen, worthy and to affirm our desired self-image. Like the way your brain naturally slots in to order the cause and effect of the latest fall-out you've had with someone, fashioning you into the possibly aggrieved, always righteous, protagonist, while your adversary becomes the wrong and nefarious. Basically, the voice that, incidentally, always tells you you're right, and maybe Patricia shouldn't have done that thing. In the same way it is important for us to be able to critically engage with these personal and meta-narratives that shape our impressions of the world around us, it is important for our children to develop the tools to do this also.

This is because, when we break the symbols and archetypes down, it reveals more about our unconscious self, our weaknesses and insecurities then it does those we wish to pigeonhole and define as a result. The cowboy itself is a short hand for liberal, Western democracies and how cultural engineers shape their time and place as global forces. The cowboy represents European colonialism and we as viewers are invited to celebrate it, and all that it stands for, in cinematic emblem. Its 'Other' – the figure of the 'Red Indian', as constructed by early modern cinema – exists not in and of itself, but to affirm Western identity; it is the wilful and justified target for American bullets and angst. It acts to prop up the identity of the cowboy and American exceptionalism, and to camouflage a whole host of social anxieties regarding American imperialism. It serves no other purpose than to contrast and attribute meaning to the good, worthy and triumphant. The 'Red Indian' is the inverted mirror for Western imperialism, it tells you everything you need to know about Empire.

Indeed, we know the history of what we now call America far precedes Western imperialism, and time itself exists outside of the beginning and end we fashion it into to conform to our own needs and wants as attempted script writers of history and meaning. Who determines where this narrative slice of time starts, what events are foregrounded and which are forgotten, and ultimately where it ends – holds a lot of power.

So, the 'Red Indian' is our collective Patricia and if we pay careful enough attention, we may see that our issues with her are likely a figment of our imagination, and that this reveals more about ourselves and our own insecurities then it does about Patricia herself. How difficult is it to overturn these narratives we self-placate with, and how much do we depend on them both in the everyday and throughout the course of our lives..?

The binary symbols of the standard, or normative cowboy, versus the Indigenous Other, have at best a tenuous claim to reality and are crafted to reassure the viewer by providing a simple moral code of virtue and goodness which acts as a smoke screen for the death and destitution American history has left in its wake. Ultimately, these metanarratives are stories humanity tells itself to disburden itself from national trauma.

[Director's notes: POV, The Muslim Mum? As Muslim mothers it is important for us to understand this often deep and complex psychology because, as we will go on to analyse, these meaning making narratives cast us in a role outside of our own making. They are the chronicles through which our children will come to learn the world, and which will tell them about themselves through this cogent language of storytelling. And because ultimately, as inheritors of the faith, we know the primary and supreme Author, and the true story of man – how and why he was created and where his purpose lies. Where our value is situated and where our journey begins and ends, by Allāh's design.]

While all this may seem obvious, attempts to consolidate the liberal, secular identity and hypercapitalism as an ideology, by creating the figure of a boogie man, are relevant to us on an everyday level because of the way they metastasise from and to arenas of non-fictive, public life. That is, the two way relationship between politics and culture, and how these narratives form the basis of institutions such as media, law, health, education – erecting and consolidating systemic inequality in the very structures that govern our public lives. As Muslims, this is incisive because these are institutions we often find ourselves on the sharp end of, and these ideologies are the hymn sheets everyone is singing from – the collective melody we all have stuck in our heads…

The stories society tells itself and the narratives we feed on follow these cinematic patterns of delusion, deflection and reassurance. Socially, we create identities of monstrosity by purging ours; by projecting our own anxieties onto an empty signifier. The supposedly deviant identities which we create culturally – our monsters or Others – only serve as an ideological aid, to distract from and cleanse dominant norms and identities. If we look at how monsters have throughout literary history embodied our most subliminal fears – how they've adopted social, racial and cultural characteristics of the communities we most demonise, and how those fears, and the process of demonisation, say more about the norms of majority society than anything else.

These less obviously fictive identities – our 'real life' 'villains' – form the underbelly of the binaries which define wider society. They carry the ideological burden of supporting this egotism. And these meaning-making structures, wielded from the top down, form and consolidate damaging ideas which devalue minority communities, and breed cultural complacency. Society creates monsters because dealing with their own demons is too real and too cumbersome. And this has far reaching and insidious consequences that we may not give a lot, if any, thought to.

The Muslim as Monster

This is particularly exemplified in the shaping of the public image of the Muslim, and has worrying, often contradictory projections on the Muslim mother in particular. For globally marginalised Muslim communities, whose very identities are ideologically colonised for that single purpose – to validate the liberal, secular identity – this foments multiple material harms, structurally and socially. But it also causes a process of self-deviation in us. This happens when extrinsic manifestations of Muslim identity are in such direct contrast with what scarce intrinsic understanding we have, as contemporary living Muslims that are so removed from our scripture. When your cultural diet, and political reality, is one which renders your very identity as aberration, this impacts your most intimate self-impressions in acute and often unknown ways. And this is not reserved for the Western Muslim – as globalisation results in the converging of an elite cultural hegemony, these ideas have worldwide traction. What happens to the marginalised when we start to think of our very selves as these lurking monsters. How does it shape the Muslim psyche when our most intimate beliefs are fastidiously fashioned into alien concepts by the world around us, so constantly? Due to this wanton, ideological brutalising of the

Muslim that we see in almost all facets of public life, Islamophobia becomes an intrinsic – if unwelcome – feature of our own internal world.

While we, as minoritised people, might think we understand these damaging stereotypes and actively work to disavow them, it's the ideological paraphernalia that comes with them that will haunt our thinking and clutter our individual and collective minds. We might think we know that all races are equal, but we will denigrate symbols concomitant with cultures that are undervalued in society. We will distance ourselves from these symbols or practices, on an instinctive level, because affiliation with the 'strong' grants us greater social capital and better self-esteem. This internalised Islamophobia means we might not want to be so closely associated to symbols of Muslimness, in whatever relative form they take in our work, schools or social settings because of implicit and unconscious biases we have absorbed from society at large. This can mean anything in any given context – for those in secular spaces, the notion of praying itself might be imbued in shame, for those in more Muslim majority or Muslim friendly spaces, there is still an inverse correlation between 'Muslimness' and legitimacy that will mean we will always try to err on the side of secularism to appear reasonable, rational and more affable – both to ourselves and others. Code-switching becomes a natural part of our social survival. It also means we might use secular logic and reasoning to legitimise Islamic belief as, as we've discussed, it is the very quality of faith and obedience to Allāh which is most stigmatised. Therefore, we must dress it up in the presentable suit of rationalism and dialect – we must add eternal caveats to seem reasonable and ethically sound and mature. Due to the macro political climate, as well as the micro psychological nuances we ourselves carry, the moral rectitude Islam embodies becomes symbolic shorthand for a kind of social immorality according to the information structures that govern our thinking.

When we look at the Muslim as Monster trope – arguably the most dominant national and global archetype – we are able to discern how the empty symbol of the Muslim identity absorbs a whole host of deep rooted issues in majority society through cultural, media and political representations. The conceptual Muslim in public imagination serves to cleanse dominant norms and identities, by acting as a sponge for society's most acute worries. The Muslim acts as a leveller to simplify these complexities and pacify wider society by providing a supposedly inverted mirror image of themselves. If there is a big bad Muslim around the corner, we are no longer fixated on the issues concerning ourselves, which require emotional and intellectual labour, and for which we don't always have all the answers.

And anti-Muslim hatred, and the acceptability it carries in wider society, is a racist's dream – it is a catharsis for those who can camouflage their bigotry under the guise of rationalism, under the vapid 'Islam is not a race' banner. It affords them the privileges of being openly, vocally and 'legitimately' hateful. It carries the unspoken hate that society cannot get away with expressing; it is a patchwork which adopts the frustrations of all the more 'illegitimate' forms of racial hatred. Because it is predicated on the idea of Muslims having the gall to be actively different – to *choose* to be 'foreign' – it is the ultimate crime in the eyes of those who are so uncomfortable with the 'Other'. Islamophobia is an emboldened hate which invites an additional fervour; Muslims as the ultimate outliers, become emblematic of every 'other' – they absorb all the undesirable characteristics created in our collective minds from the detritus of our own ego. This irrational hatred masquerading as rationalism becomes a shorthand for intellectualism itself, that right-wing figures borrow from to appear erudite and claim intellectually credibility. Tellingly, Islamophobia is also entirely incongruous and inconsistent as an ideology; this is why at Islamophobic rallies the average man or woman who has been whipped up into a rabid, anti-Muslim frenzy, is entirely incoherent, illogical and unable to articulate their apparent world view.

Indeed, Islamophobic, fascist riots that took place across the UK in the summer of 2024, following the false claim that a Muslim man was responsible for child-stabbings[xv], is just one of the many real life fictions which are symbolic of a hate which is entirely baseless, illogical and predicated on outright lies and paranoia. It is effectively our most subconscious fear personified through a racism that is openly expressed through policy, media discourse, institutional foot prints and culture. Despite this obfuscation of it, Islamophobia bears all the hallmarks of the racism it denies itself to be – it's a hate based on a 'racialised' identity and depends upon a subordination of a culture, entrenched by systematic and structural inequality.[xvi] And I use the term racialised here and throughout the book, because white Muslims are subject to the same nationalistic and xenophobic bigotry where they wouldn't be if they were not so visibly Muslim – be they 'revert' Muslims or Muslims that hail from Muslim Europe. The concept of "whiteness" that many claim they are fighting to defend is entirely socially constructed, in the same way all racial identities are, despite 'whiteness' being framed as a 'non-race', or as though it is the standard way of being. Ultimately, Islamophobia has passed the dinner table, lunch room and breakfast bar test – it is the thinking man's bigotry which is actively rewarded in society in how it affords its advocates social, cultural and financial capital. Careers have been forged, and clout has been afforded to those brave and outspoken enough to add to the chorus of hate against arguably one of the most marginalised communities that exists.

Conversely, we could say an individual's Islamophobia is a reflection of so much more; we could use it as a measure of its owners insecurity and general sense of unease with difference, and their own opinion of themselves. By extension, each culture has its own flavour of Islamophobia which reflects its collective weaknesses. The distinctly French brand of Islamophobia which exposes its own discomfort – as the coveted birth place of secular democracy – in using the freedoms it fought religion to bear, to protect the religious rights of those it colonised. It could be argued that British Islamophobia evolved from an embryonic anti-South Asian hate – following one of the first recognised waves of mass immigration, which came from the subcontinent – and the very specific bigotry this gave rise to. Indeed, one of the most prominent racial slurs quintessential to the UK, which itself is tellingly used as a catch-all profanity, is aimed at those of Pakistani descent. Modern notions of Islamophobia in Britain still carry those same anti-South Asian hues, despite the Muslim population growing increasingly diverse, and Muslims from other ethnicities facing additional racism there. American Islamophobia has its own roots in anti-African American sentiment, given how domestic forms of Islam developed – Islamophobia beginning in the civil rights era was inextricably linked to America's own uniquely abhorrent history of anti-black racism. The commonality in all these examples, and many more, is these are racialised, working class communities, overwhelmingly from economically disadvantaged backgrounds, which hints at where some of this anti-Muslim hate emanates from – certainly even in some Muslim corners of the globe, there is undoubtedly some convergence in class and anti-Islamic sentiment, which illustrates the underlying tensions, and biases, these bigotries are born from. The sum effect of this being, of course, that depending where we as Muslim mums sit on a spectrum of class, race and nationality – the prejudices we are subject to are likely to take on different hues.

So, let's break down how the Muslim in popular imagination tells us everything we need to know about those social anxieties at large, today.

The fictive, symbolic figure of the 'Muslim as barbaric' is used in contrast to enhance rational, secular humanism – the post-Enlightenment philosophy which claims to privilege man's thinking function, and science, above all else. We look at how Muslim governments, tribes and other cultural groups are constantly deemed as neolithic, barefooted, cave-dwelling, and how this is further down the line of 'civilised', and how that in turn makes Western secularists feel refined, polished – worthy of the role and title of coloniser. The "Muslim as rapist" to divert from issues concerning sexual morality in wider society. The idea that Muslim men are inherently sexually predatory we see time and time again in domestic and global media, which helps to supress our worries about sexual mores, and the increased gamification of dating and relationships excelled by dating apps and social media in the new digitised age. The "Muslims as death cult" to relieve the intellectual crisis centring on secular notions of after-life – or lack thereof – that may give rise to a lack of meaning, direction or purpose, questioning the very notion of mortality. The very idea that Muslims may work towards an afterlife, or by extension value their *shaheed*[19], triggers something in secular imagination so deep, a rebuking that makes evident the feeling that our faith and notions of after-life must be intellectually colonised also. The "Muslim as terrorist", serving to distract from the existential crisis facing Western imperialism; if Western democracies are the ultimate symbols of statehood and citizenship, if the very political identity of the West is based upon the hero-worship of democracy, then through the fictive identity of the Muslim they can purge the complexities that arise in a post-Brexit/Trump world. The insecurities that undermine those democratic systems and processes they hold on to so dearly need no longer be the focus of political attention when the Muslim is there to adopt those flaws. And of course, the "Muslim as stateless", to compound citizenship, identity and belonging at a time where public disquiet around national borders and identity is most frantic. This idea that Muslims are always lurking at those borders, threatening the very stability of the fortress of Europe and the American Dream is the ultimate affront to constitutional identities, and to a populism that seeks to preserve a fictive

---

[19] Martyrs

history of racial purity. The cultural mythology of the Muslim as borderless, both individually and collectively, embalms the majority against issues of individual and national identity – and the nation state itself – at a time when it is most confounded. These issues belie the laughably dramatic and hackneyed 'clash of civilisation' narrative that so much of Western imperialism depends upon – both in its ideology and its military, social and political actions. It is also why the logical conclusion for the Muslim is always death – be it in the politics that governs modern warfare, or the racism we individually face on the street – the threat is always death.

In order to avoid holding up a mirror to itself, mainstream society – dictated by political powers and elite consensus – chooses to distance itself from these issues by projecting them onto the figurative Muslim.[xvii] And of course these issues of crisis are heightened and felt more acutely as Western liberalism faces its greatest challenge to date, as its relevance and dominance is questioned and it's economic and cultural influence wanes. The linear idea of progress on which secular humanism is built upon and on which it depends, is eroding as we face an apocalyptic future of climate emergency and its own political impotence. There is no neat, reassuring finale to the story that secular humanism has lulled itself to sleep on, this is not the end of history as we know it, and we have not reached an apex of civilisation – we may in fact be some way past crescendo. And this is why it is doubling down hard on the conceptual Muslim, to avoid facing a whole host of issues regarding the values that underpin it. This is the cause of the heightened, increasingly irrational and worrying Islamophobia we see in many corners of the globe.

And so, while majority identities are debating the unbearable lightness of being, adherents to Islam are living the unbearable politicisation of being Muslim. 'The Muslim' is a narrative device wielded by the most powerful to subdue the population at large. It is the story of our time, and a narrative so pervasive that not only does it shape national and foreign policy, primarily and fundamentally, these policies shape the conceptual Muslim. It plays itself out in media, policy and arts – through the news we consume, the laws that govern us and the media we build our basic cultural assumptions and values over.

While this is, as we've mentioned, overwhelmingly instigated by authorities that benefit politically, there are cottage-industry versions which profiteer from fear pedalling, a notoriously lucrative industry from which institutions and careers will be built and forged. During the onset of the pandemic, when public anger and anxiety was redirected away from Muslims, and we saw a slight shift from Islamophobic to anti-vax talking points, many high-profile shock jockeys followed this profitable pipeline, repositioning themselves as defenders of bodily, not religious, freedom. Indeed, to keep up with their old habits of Islamophobia, there was a conscious effort to conflate Muslims with the fear and disease of the pandemic as was evident in the way media stories concerning Covid were so disproportionately illustrated by images of Muslims.[xviii] A rare sight to see the media outlets scurry together to ensure Muslim (over)representation, indeed, the exhausting of stock images of visible Muslims was almost quite heartening. Then, and now, Islamophobia continues to be incredibly financially and publicly rewarding, with funding of far-right, anti-Muslim think tanks often purposefully obscured, through transatlantic links, to hide this patent fact. It is ready and poised to take on the shape of any impending social anxiety and doom – and parenting against this backdrop means we will be more vulnerable to the ideological gymnastics that arise as a result.

[Director's notes: Not everyday "The Muslim as Other"; while the themes we deconstruct through this chapter highlight a very specific narrative ploy, it is important to remember that this ploy is not propagated, supported, nor accepted by everyone or even all the time. This much is evident in the millions of instances of truly wholesome relationships and interactions we are blessed with from within and outside of the community. And it is evident in world events like the 2022 FIFA World Cup, hosted in Qatar, and in which social media coverage of Muslims was overwhelmingly positive, despite legacy media, and the billionaire press barons who steer it, labouring to achieve the opposite. Proximity theory – which states that human prejudice erodes when we are at proximity to those we alienise, and that social, spatial and cultural distance breeds hostility and contempt – demonstrates as much. **Allāh** *tells us Islam will be strange, and part of navigating that truth – as a Muslim mum – is understanding the social, political and cultural manifestations of that strange. And part of that manifestation is the tragic consequence of increasingly stratified countries ruled by elites that are economically and ideologically dependent upon an underclass. Muslims, for social, economic and geo-political reasons, are often conveniently placed to assume the role of that villainised underclass. The powerful will always want to remain in and preserve their power, and often we fall victim to this endeavour, and this is one element of the strange that we inhabit as a faith group– as people with a faith that grants us the dignity to do so.]*

Human Rights, Muslims Wrong

In the carte blanche industry of perpetual wars, fuelled by a propaganda machine built upon the paradox of democracy promotion in Muslim majority countries, the very concept of citizenship in particular evades the Muslim. On the benign end of the scale, this applies to the sheer media hysteria around the 'Muslim Vote' in the UK, in July 2024, and the parallel conversation across the Atlantic, aimed at American Muslim voters of the same year, expressing discomfort in voting for the Democrats. What underlies and exemplifies some of this political sentiment is the idea that Muslims, and indeed other racialised communities, cannot be 'working class' – there is little solidarity with marginalised communities amongst popular labour movements – or indeed middle class as we go on to explore. On the far more malignant end, the idea of civic rights and identity evading Muslims is evident for the hundreds of thousands killed in Iraq, the lives taken in the twenty-year war against Afghanistan and drone warfare targeting Pakistanis. If the Muslim state is the failed state, in need of 'correction', then the very construct of civic identity does not apply to Muslim citizens. It is a breath-takingly arrogant necropolotics, a deciding of who is worthy of death, which is inherently blasphemous in nature.

We, as a global population – Muslim and none – are able to justify indiscriminate killing of Muslim life: because the notion of 'civilian life' that is so sacred to international law is not extended to the Muslim itself. This is true of the conflict impacting Muslims in Sudan, the ethnic cleansing of Uyghurs and Rohingyas and the torture and killing of Syrians. The lofty commitment to the principle of human rights does not extend to Muslim rights, just like the commitment to anti-racist sentiment often stops short of Muslims. Social panic does not extend to loss of Muslim life, in fact, conversely, it is instigated by the very preservation and propagation of Muslim life. This fact is exemplified by domestic as well as foreign policy, as we will go on to interrogate, but also by the media and political uproar concerning the many dignified and justified demonstrations and marches around the world in support of Gaza in 2023 and 2024. The idea that the status quo of the killing of Muslims should be disrupted appeared to cause more concern than those killings themselves.

So warping is the idea that majority society is wronged by the nefarious, plotting Muslim that it creates the kind of cognitive dissonance in which violent acts against Muslims are at best minimised, and at worst justified, by virtue of how unrighteous and inhuman its target is – think of the tragic and incomprehensible loss of life in Gaza which the world didn't deem worthy of an accurate death count. The same situation in Gaza which exposed a hardwiring of Islamophobia in American evangelical culture – their default identity appears to be based on anti-Muslim sentiment which sees them taking up the cause of Israel's genocide with an alarming sense of enthusiasm.

Muslims, ironically, are so deviant and inherently racist, we are ourselves deserving of being on the receiving end of such deviant racism. This has become an convenient truism for the Kleptocracy's that profit so keenly from wars in Muslim lands, who claim to be fighting bigotry and intolerance, while using the very weapons of bigotry and intolerance to do so. And this is where the amorphous nature of Islamophobia is such a useful tool – socially, politically and geo-politically. When the very nature of 'Muslimness', and what within that identity is constituted as dangerous and threatening to hegemonic notions of 'Western' identity, remains amorphous, it creates a convenient elasticity which can be used to justify any kind of military action. When you base the conceptual identity of The Muslim on your own fears, it is shaped timely and accordingly. This is why Israel is able to cut off water supply and deny entry of food and aid to an entire population of people, because the danger exists in the woman, child, the home, school, mosque – entire human and social structures. This is also why we can justify the use of nuclear weapons against a ghettoised, forty-one kilometre long strip, one of the most densely populated areas on earth, and within which half the population are children. It remains politically expedient to have a whole class of people ripe for demonisation, to evoke the spectre that exists in all of our minds – a kind of flat pack monster, ready to be erected in ways that benefit the political elite.

What's odiously hypocritical of those cheerleaders of war and genocide amongst the political right, and what exemplifies the underlying assumption that Muslim families are the *opposite* of life affirming – is that many of these conservative political and media figures have been voted in on the ticket of preserving the sacred institution of the family and home, while advocating for its very dissolution in the Muslim world. In Gaza in particular we see families entirely dismembered by the onslaught, and whole blood lines wiped out. We also see the gross exoneration of Israel's actions by those citing the very fact that an estimated half of the Gazan population are children – as though Israel has benevolently "allowed" and "accepted" this fact of Muslim life, and that the fact itself attests to Muslim's dangerously conspiring to... exist? That this demographic statistic is crudely referenced to justify military intervention, as part of inherently racist 'overpopulation' claims, underscores the very point about the questioning of Muslim right to life, legitimacy and space on earth. Particularly when we juxtapose this conversation with the social anxiety, and conversations more generally, around declining fertility rates in the West. These wars instigated by the West make multiple claims, fighting on multiple plains – geographical, historical and metaphysical; as though it is their role to bestow a right to exist.

If this book is constructed around the Muslim mum, then what sits at its nucleus is the Muslim child. These are our children that are at the brutal, culling end of this ideological warfare instigated by colonial powers – our children in Sudan, in China, Iraq, Yemen. And these injustices need to be fought, in every way possible, by all of us.

The visual standard of being Muslim

If the Muslim represents the absolute antithesis of the civic individual, the noble and dignified human, then the monster becomes more subhuman, and worthy of more extremes, than we can possibly imagine. Again, this is made explicit with this harrowing genocide in Gaza, which itself was aided and abetted by the Islamophobia industry, and the visual culture it exemplifies. While colonial violence has historically been un – or poorly-documented, witnessing the execution of it in real time is nothing short of earth shattering. The images and video footage of Muslim suffering are so severe, and the statistics, civic journalism and anecdotal information from aid agencies paint a picture of violence hitherto unknown in modern warfare, creating the deadliest and most destructive conflict in the twenty-first century. And this is despite how much the image has itself shaped intervention in conflict zones historically. How images of suffering in pre-digital contexts has led to tokenistic action, and how the culture of the spectacle has impacted foreign policy; in a world reduced to surfaces, the image is imbued with much cultural significance. In conflicts such as those in Syria, Iraq and Sudan, where we see such distressing images emerge, there is not even the tokenistic rewarding of spectatorship that governs war reporting and photojournalism. These images have no impact on the world at large. Because both those civilians bearing witness to, reporting and being on the receiving end of such violence are not deemed worthy of either the 'objective' role of legitimate reporters, nor the humanity that deserves preserving, and which would demand condemnation of such senseless, brutal violence.

It is clear, we are visually trained to accept, maybe even expect, the brutalising of Muslims as the epitome of 'foreign other' for the comfort, safety and security of the Western world. So we see that the genocide in Gaza, and indeed much of the occupation that preceded it and the forever wars adjacent to it, are facilitated by the lessening and 'cheapening' of Muslim life itself. The lens through which much of the world sees Muslim life means war crimes are anywhere on a spectrum of acceptable, quotidian, invisible and necessary.

The idea of Muslim as less-than in visual narratives has also meant a double standard in the visual reporting of human catastrophe by mainstream Western media outlets themselves. While many consciously chose to refrain from broadcasting video and imagery of Ukrainian refugees in a commendable attempt to maintain their dignity, this has never been the case for Muslims, whom the camera lens perceives with a clinical distance, and with detached sentiment. The threshold for Muslim suffering is much higher due to ongoing dehumanisation which will always frame Muslim pain as something to survey and behold. What exemplifies this, is the callous and morally bankrupt cartoons, often in French satirist newspapers and magazines, mocking Muslims even when withstanding a genocide.[xix] Newspapers and magazines that would themselves object to Muslims on the basis of a perceived ethical inferiority unironically expose their own gaping moral cavity.

If the retaining of humanity for those racialised as "white" is to censor images of suffering and displacement, then what does it mean that we must share the most unspeakable images of Muslims to prove their own humanity and in a futile attempt to provoke action? Why do we applaud journalists for their inaction in spectating on disaster, yet ignore the bravery of the citizen journalism unfolding in Muslim countries, documenting their subjugation, against the most horrific conditions. What does that mean about the standards of humanity we set for Muslims, where we place agency, and how much we value Muslim blood? The fact remains we are trained, once again, on an instinctual, visual level, to normalise Muslim death and suffering as an inevitable part of our backdrop. And that extraordinary Muslim acts of bravery are secondary to Western spectatorship and inaction.

This visual training means the global colonial atrocities that we are now seeing reported through citizen journalism hold a mirror up to the wider world. Those of us who have experienced marginalisation – the 'underside' of the binary – see ourselves in the colonised, and those who identify with the powerful – the dominant identity – see themselves in the colonial settler force. Those of us that are marginalised possess a fear that we would ever come close to being as inhumane, and blinded by hate, as those oppressive regimes are in their bombardment and massacre. What motivates the powerful across the world is the fear that they will taste marginalisation and all that comes with it. What powers us as the marginalised, is to prevent further human suffering, and what is behind the actions of those that dominate is to insulate themselves from cruelty they appear to identify as universally human. Part of what makes these atrocities verbally disabling is that it has brought up the spectre of a value system we have been normalising for so long, it has exorcised to the surface some of the ugliest features of humanity that we long thought were buried but which have been operating undetected for so long. Along with other valuable lessons, those Muslims that have endured, and continue to endure, oppressive and colonial regimes have taught us to be cognisant of our own internal narratives – the very language by which we interpret meaning, develop values and adopt and enact our worldview.

This unfortunate visual standard which normalises Muslim suffering has been adopted by Muslim communities themselves – as is evident in the lack of restraint, and visual exploitation carried out by a majority of Muslim aid agencies in fundraising campaigns, and which trickles down to the everyday Muslim who unquestioningly shares images of Muslims in disaster zones, and in other vulnerable positions such as receiving food parcels and other necessities denied to them through circumstance. As Muslim parents, for whom charity is a core element of our faith, we are taking our children on fundraising drives, amongst this moral dissymmetry. This trend is in direct contradiction to religious edicts which clearly state charity is an act of mercy and compassion from God for the donor, more so than the recipient. The hierarchy is inverted in Muslim theology, and having the opportunity to distribute our wealth to those momentarily in less fortunate circumstances is considered a blessing for those in the position to do so. Yet we are so used to Muslim suffering being turned into a kind of performance in the act of charity and the story of saviour-hood, we have willingly perpetuated this perverse optical code. Perhaps this explains the inaction from Muslim governments themselves – we have become desensitised to Muslim suffering on an intracommunity level too.

It is worth exploring how these visual imbalances in media and politics sit against a broader artistic and visual culture which shapes Muslim identity for spectatorship. Indeed, the visual depiction of the Muslim in Western art and culture has its own historical quirks that impact the Muslim woman and mum in particular. Dictated by the fetishism of orientalism, artistic representations of Muslim men, women and Islamic culture have themselves been a reflection of Western intrigue and frustration with the Other. And while technology and cultural narratives have themselves sophisticated, the underlying anthropological sentiment has crystalised in much of the imagery that has come to define how Muslims are presented to visual audiences in Western art today.

This lens of orientalising and otherising is particularly focused on the Muslim woman. We see this in contemporary art forms, which use the tired, postmodern trope of objectification as a tool to de-objectify in art and photography concerning

Muslim women. The unbelievably crude and conceited visual code of juxtaposing Muslim women with 'modern' objects such as bikes (those wheels again…), boom boxes and other paraphernalia to make a supposedly subversive point about a usually secular artist's ability to conceive of these women as more than just objects is an entire trope which deserves unpacking in itself. Similarly, trends emanating from internet culture, like the hackneyed 'then' and 'now'-ing of Muslim countries using images of women from pre-Islamic iterations of modern day Muslim states with contemporary photographs, are also based on asinine thinking. Used as a tool by far right commentators, it has become a visual shorthand to demonstrate the supposedly regressive nature of Islam, and has the kind of immediate impact that delights politically immature thinkers who conflate modernity with Western ideals. Showing images of bare legged Muslim women in a 1950s, secular pre-Islamic state versus those nationals in hijab in contemporary day is not the 'own' people think it is. Both of these prementioned trends are equally offensive, but the former prides itself in being a 'knowing', 'conscious', self-reflexive interpretation, which again results in this perennial congratulating of artist and audience in continually 'rediscovering' and thinking 'better' of the

Muslim woman. They attribute the very idea of Muslim women being more than just insentient beings to their own supposed benevolence and intellect. We, as Muslim women, are effectively reduced and flattened into a symbol of passive accessory in someone else's gauche and self-indulgent story. While this may seem a niche trend, we know that concepts, themes and tropes in "high" culture filter so acutely down into mainstream and popular culture – and we know that the visual climate through which Muslim women are referencing themselves becomes incredibly alienating and punishing as a result.

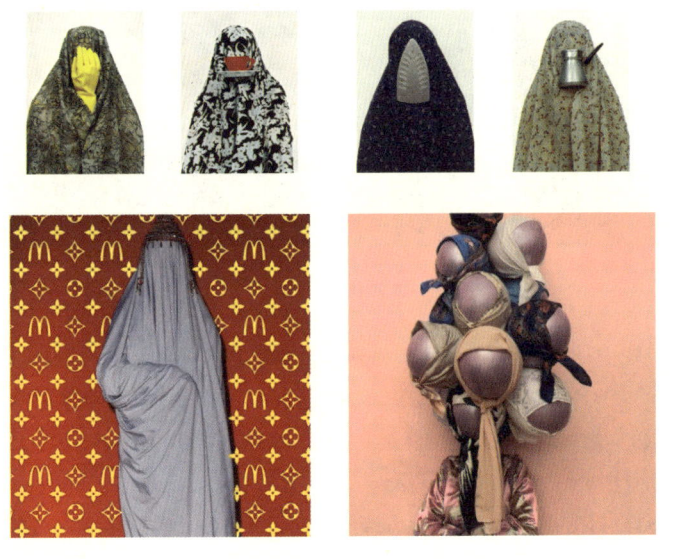

Perhaps the most comical iteration of anti-Muslim visual trends is how AI is used by far-right groups to depict the Muslim. It is both predictable and depressing that these new tools of creativity and imagination are denigrated to unequivocally perpetuate age old biases. Despite the limitless potential of AI, many can't see it beyond its ability to act as a kind of crude Microsoft paint for their racist imagination... Nonetheless, it has unlocked the imaginative potential of a class of people with the most myopic world view. You might ask what the world's most powerful intelligence tool can do when in the hands of arguably some of the most inept minds, and the answer would be nothing surprising, really.

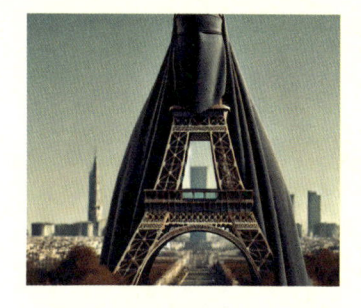

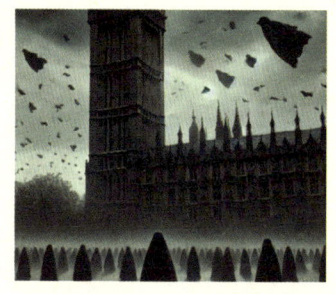

Like a racist fever dream, resultant depictions of Muslims in AI art propagated by these xenophobic groups and individuals are comically exaggerated and restricted to old boorish tropes. These modern day Monets depict us either entirely dehumanised, in our many and less distinguishable, or background fodder to a hero-worshiping fallacy of white supremacy. These works are so potent and emotionally charged, it's almost possible to hear the racist tears that powered the AI engines to make them.

As younger artists of Muslim heritage, who have more digitally imaginative tools at their disposable, and are therefore less indebted to the material imbalances in our aesthetic environment, are increasingly taking control of their visual narratives, it is likely Gen Alpha Muslims at least will live in a more balanced visual landscape. An emerging trend of futuristic, sci-fi and fantasy styles of art that this change is giving rise to is both refreshing and heartening to see. This Muslim Avant Garde art and the potential direction it will take in the future is certainly something to be hopeful about, both in how it does not compromise on Islamic principles, centres the Islamic gaze, and decouples visual representations of Muslims from the historic negative stereotypes we have erstwhile been connected to. It speaks of an ability to imagine a Muslim future unhindered by the stereotypes that have hitherto restricted it.

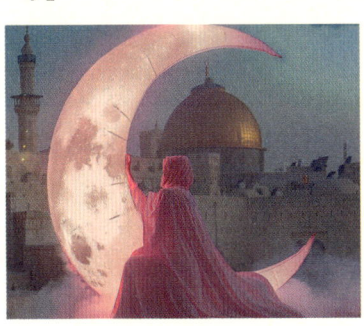

The paradox of punishing Muslims for agency

In how the world responded to Gaza we see the sinister paradox in which Muslims are punished for the human-defining quality of agency, and restricted through the qualifying feature of their God-given right of freedom. And this against a global backdrop in which we appear to have to ask permission to be Muslim, and then adapt how that Muslimness expresses itself for others' comfort. To shape the borders of our religious identity according to others' sensitivities and tolerance.

Gaza is a compelling example because when exploring modern Muslim motherhood, it simply cannot be ignored. Both for the sheer other-worldly levels of heroism mums in Gaza have so graciously embodied, for the many beautiful souls of mothers, children, fathers, grandfathers…that are elevated to the status of shaheed, and how we as Muslim mums will carry the grief and pain of their suffering in life-altering ways. There is simply no contemporary event that has had such an impact on the collective DNA of Muslim mothers, than this world-changing atrocity, with all the trauma of a collective nightmare. It has exposed a fear that mothers hold on such a cellular level. The fear of having to leave our young children unprotected on earth amidst their continuing dehumanisation, suffering and violence. Or the equally harrowing alternative of bearing witness to your child's soul leaving it's body before you have to face a chilling lifetime without them. For Muslim mums this is a material reality – made possible by the vilification of our very identity.

We consider agency and volition as key human characteristics both in secular and non-secular thinking. Enlightenment ideals, such as supposed equality and liberty, which dictate a secular humanism that has shaped much of the modern world, are based on the premise of man as rational agent. And Islamically we know Allāh gave Adam choice – as something that discerns man above jinn and angel. If the Muslim is the inverted human – then how does the world react to Muslim agency itself? And what does this mean for Muslim mothers, for whom parental agency is an equally defining characteristic?

When we are intent on framing Muslim identity as a tortured inversion of mainstream sentiments, then agency becomes a punishable offence for Muslims. Muslims in the context of Britain and America, for example, are subject to punitive measures for agency itself – our choice to *be* Muslim, to choose the 'foreign' identity of Muslim, as previously discussed, is something liberal sensitivities can only withstand through pinched and upturned noses. This punishment of agency of Muslims in the West extends, of course, to political agency – what's often deemed our ultimate evil. The very notion of a Muslim as anything other than politically conformist hurts our common sense of decency – we want to see it as deviant and criminal. This denigration of Muslim agency is despite the fact that secular thinking cites their very dislike of Islam and Muslims due to the lack of apparent agency in religion. We are lauded because we cannot do what we *want* and abide by a supposedly restrictive religious code.

The indelible stain on history that is Israel's conduct in Gaza, demonstrates the ultimate punishing of Muslim agency. Israel feels it has the right to choose who lives, who dies, to deny Gazans in the absolute sense any agency. It dresses up this heinous ideology and abhorrent acts in a passive language which posits Israel's active genocide onto the Palestinian. Media headlines concerning the genocide across the Western globe (including those that abominably state 'lives found ended'...) took the passive voice to its absolute limit to absolve Israel of any crimes.[xx] It posits the responsibility of the genocide firmly on the very people it is ethnically cleansing. It paints Palestinian victimhood as active aggressor, reframes the inaction of being killed as the cause and punishment for Muslim agency.

We see less lethal, but very worrying trends in policy in countries such as France which also take on this paradoxical approach to Muslim will. In the denying of the hijab, abaya, and modest swimwear in varying contexts, we see a gracious removing of civil liberties and freedom in order to celebrate those very qualities themselves. Because Muslim freedom is a nullified concept – we cannot be Muslim and be free according to mainstream sentiment. These policies are designed to undress Muslim women – and are predicated on a warped sense of agency which prioritises Western ideas of liberty and freedom. Denying Muslim women movement, choice and agency because…Islam has apparently denied us this? France in a constant one upmanship with the spectre of Islam it has created from its own racist imagination, and colonial hang-ups…

This is entirely consistent in the way Muslim women are used as fodder for wars and the narratives that justify them. We are simultaneously sexualised and desexualised to suit whatever narrative is most advantageous to the military-industrial complex and the corporation of war. In one instance, a lack of overt sexuality in Muslim women is used to justify invasion – as though our apparent need for sexual liberation is dependent on oil acquisition. And in more recent iterations, where the goal is simply to exterminate all life, we see how IDF soldiers pose again and again with Gazan's women's garments, denoting an apparent culpability simply for possessing clothing that is sexualised. In one instance, sexuality is used as a measure of liberation, and in another it is imposed upon as and cited as proof of our degeneracy and cause for genocide.

In Gaza, we see the logical extension of denying Muslim's parental agency in particular – Muslim mums have no say or right to protect their children from their own needless and callous murders at the hands of a genocidal regime. The Israeli government, and those governments in the West that fund them, have robbed Muslim mothers of their very children's lives. As Muslim women we recognise and feel this in our very core, every time we are confronted with the crimes of this supremacist ideology.

Indeed Muslim agency itself is seen as so degenerate that it can only be attributable through acts of terror. The modern idiom of 'innocent until proven Muslim' rings true here – when we see violence carried out by individuals who identify – or are identified as – Muslim it becomes an act of terror, yet any other faith, and that agency towards terror is nullified.

It's important to note here that agency, is exactly where the fruits of our deeds lie. Our crowning feature – and the key determiner of our path to Jannah[20] – is in this choice. There is no compulsion in religion, and of course all of us have come to Islam with a full and beautiful sense of agency and volition. So while we are often publicly ridiculed simply for the very perception of a lack of agency, and contrarily punished for our agency in choosing our faith, it is the will with which we submit to Allāh, and fulfil our obligations as Muslims, that will grant us the most reward in our eternal abode. Despite mainstream denigration and punishment of Muslim agency, we are elevated through it, and in it Allāh has posited our reward.

How the Muslim Mother is framed

So, how does this discursive tsunami impact the embattled Muslim mother? We know that social anxieties are played out most acutely in

---

20 Heaven

the language of the family and home, and often the policies which govern it, and institutions that neighbour it. This is why when, for example, society is shocked into a panic concerning obesity – and general health concerning modern living standards – we see policy proposals to penalise this in schools, grant free FitBits, tax fried chicken shops in school vicinities, a discursive storm that rains down on the home. The same is true of Islam and how the Muslim family becomes the projected social site, and proposed policy cure, for many of those anxieties.

In this strange and tumultuous time in political and cultural history, the underlying tensions and anxieties we see simmering are linked to the idea of "creeping shariah" – a perceived overt and covert attack on the very identity, autonomy and rights of white, majority populations in much of Europe and North America. The very threat is deemed as existential both through the wider discourse, and how it is sometimes interpreted individually on the street. Exacerbating this is the sharp decline in fertility rates in post-industrialised countries, leading to what many right-wing thinkers bemoan as 'The Great Replacement'. This sentiment – which has a lot of cultural traction – mourns the discrepancy between the rate of reproduction in often Muslim, always globally southern, nations which are on a continued upward trajectory. If the coloniser's greatest fear is to be colonised, then a rise in the world's Muslims continues to be a great source of concern both domestically and internationally.

This is because the threat is also perceived within the very state itself – with a rise in ethnic minorities, and by extension Muslims, in white majority countries themselves (countries that we have conveniently forgotten were colonisers in many of these immigrants' lands, in a unique cause/effect blindness that occurs when we are reviewing geopolitics…). This leads to a kind of social paranoia concerning potential 'fifth columns', the enemy within, a foreign insurgence, and various other Star Wars-themed fever dreams. This fear does not, interestingly, filter down to immigrants racialised as white – for example European immigrants to Western countries are often perceived unproblematically in civic and national terms. Often even census counts do not register the race of white immigrants beyond second and third generations; as though their natural absorption into the country is presumed in a way that it is not for racialised communities. Laughably, this subconscious fear sometimes finds expression in very lucid and explicit ways – with a more recent example being a staunch, Biblically worded speech made by a member of the House of Lords in Great Britain, which claimed of Muslims, that the "radicals will take us over through the power of the womb" [xxi] While this evoked a strange, warm feeling for many of us, radiating sinisterly from the midriff area (reminiscent, almost, of a Power Rangers/Telly Tubbies kind of cross over...) it is always telling when political figures say the quiet bits out loud, particularly in the government buildings we fund.

Much of this is projected in headlines in right-wing, and increasingly centrist, Western media concerning Muslim's burdening health, education and housing systems in countries they are legitimate tax payers, and cultural and social contributors in. Muslims are also centred in the defining political issue of our time – immigration to Western countries, indeed, many argue anti-immigrant sentiment is a proxy for anti-Muslim sentiment.[xxii] Most of which implicates the symbolically passive role of the Muslim mum as reproducer. The Muslim mother represents the cradle of Muslim civilisation in many ways – if Muslim life is so vilified, where does the bringer-of that life sit in the court of public and political opinion? She sits with all the gravity of colonising suspicion and endeavour you might expect.

The idea of the Muslim woman is intrinsically linked to that of the Muslim mother and wife in public imagination – the Muslim woman poses an imagined threat on the basis of her potential to procreate; to be an active accessory to this great replacement. Despite all the lip service regarding female autonomy and liberation, it remains sardonically true that Muslim women are conceived as a kind of undetachable accessory in the eyes of those nations that claim to be fighting the hardest for our liberation. The Muslim woman and mother, therefore, is implicated in both explicit and implicit ways when we speak of supposed Muslim villainy.

None of us are strangers to this cold politicisation of the female, Muslim identity, and her capacity to mother as central to that. Fortunately for politicians, the veiled Muslim woman, with its ideologically pregnable history, is the perfect rhetorical shorthand for 'Them', to contrast and bolster the insular and tribal 'Us'. Coupled with the political elasticity of the Muslim identity more generally, and it means as a demographic, Muslim women have an electoral store of value akin to gold to demagogues and the broader political class alike. And so, we become a coin heavy with reassurance, traded most frequently during election cycles and opportune news days to those desperate to appeal to or distract the electoral majority. We are accustomed to expecting the supposedly casual, off-hand comment about Muslim women by a suited, snake-oil selling statesman every time there is an election pending. A carefully drafted statement brainstormed off the back of a series of focus groups, feeding off of and fuelling a self-perpetuating cycle of Islamophobic sentiment which is as reliably constant, and erratically fluctuating, as the weather. Often times these Islamophobic, political sleights of hand are designed to in-group signal, and camouflage the elite, privately educated background of the speaker in question – lend them the nonchalant, common-sense, salt of the earth persona that will convince those at the ballot box that their interests are being represented. For this, the sacrificial lamb is always the Muslim woman – we are "letterboxes" and other conveniently derided things when it is politically advantageous for us to be so. The everyday nature of anti-Muslim sentiment means in the marketplace of ideas, the Muslim woman is undoubtedly the most failsafe stock for those wanting to appear relatable and electable.

The Muslim mother, in all that she represents, also forms the basis of the justification for both domestic anti-terror policy, military intervention and genocide. It is her permissive and evocative image that is summoned in faux-earnest when both politics and geopolitics calls. She carries the unique burden of being in constant need of rescuing. She is either to be saved from the evil clutches of Islam – of needing to be civilised or colonised in order to be granted freedom – or she must be written out of history for being in full grips of it; to prevent the production of future terrorists. Of being spoken for, and over, in a condescending and vain attempt to grant her a voice. Of having to be visually available and optically desirable in order to be deemed liberated. She is constantly being discussed and written about – as well as being subject to an ever increasing, self-indulgent web of 'under the veil' cultural paraphernalia – the roots of which lie in some of the earliest orientalist texts. Her framing in political terms is always paradoxically one that renders her infantile and in need of assistance but still highly instrumental – and responsible – for the Muslim men in her life.

Much of the British counter violent extremist efforts were channelled into English language classes for older Muslim mothers because they are both victim and hero to a narrative which casts the Muslim as problematic. This also exposes a kind of reduction of the Muslim female experience – while this as a policy sentiment is designed to act as a catch-all for British Muslim mothers, really it is based on perceptions of the South Asian Muslim mother, whose migratory patterns are very different to, say, Somali Muslim women, who make up an entirely different matriarchal culture – resulting in total erasure of whole Muslim communities. A fact that that goes entirely unrecognised in public discourse, and in a global diaspora discourse that erroneously, and to our own detriment, privileges Arab and South Asian models of Muslimhood.

Of course, at its most extreme this false and symbolic idea of the Muslim woman leads to actual violence and harassment that we are subject to universally, irrespective of our racial make-up – there is a marked uptick in Islamophobic hate crime against visibly Muslim women in particular following these political slips of the tongue.[xxiii] As though the inevitable cost for political purchase amongst the country's most powerful is violence towards the Muslim woman – the price politicians are willing to pay is emboldening those that are so inclined to act upon their subliminal hate. But the payout for this is often in the mundane too. For many who do not question status-quo narratives, the Muslim mum is a passive and subservient agent that simply can't help herself, in the grips of a violent ideology that is by definition a threat to her threatening children. We are only good for having babies. An irritating accessory to the villainous Muslim man. An obtrusive inconvenience in a system which privileges a flexibility enslaved to the whims of the self. Very often, particularly because of our visibility, Muslim mothers are at the coalface of this bigotry.

Muslims mums are perceived as though we are on borrowed land, in borrowed time, with a kind of expectation that suggests we must seek permission to parent. As though our presence in the ideological dimension is unwelcome, that we infringe upon even the conceptual domain of rational secularism. Our faith is often perceived with a kind of disdain that is cemented from centuries of orientalism and otherising, and which simply cannot perceive of anything outside of the neoliberal value system as being equal or worthy. It is also often met with the kind of self-centring arrogance that construes other people's life choices as an affront to their own – a judgemental predisposition that perceives totally innocuous, personal acts of Islamic worship as though they are a personal slight against themselves.

Often we feel this in the Islamophobia that hangs low and heavy in the air – in sitting opposite the teacher on parents evening, in the quiet smiling gaze we're frequently met with when discussing our children's desire for a prayer room. Or in speaking to the GP, the tight lipped, forced nod of approval when we are enquiring after the ingredients of the flu vaccine. Or with the elderly lady at the bus stop who fixes herself loudly in her seat. Sometimes, it is the presence of children – a visible reminder of those pesky and dangerous wombs, back at it again – that will attract that murmur of disapproval, spoken in the language of passive racism – tuts and eyerolls, barely heard mutterings. Sometimes it is the strained sense of tolerance, by undermining our very sense of legitimacy and questioning our ability to parent children whose default is obviously a form of liberalism that Islam sits in apparent opposition to. As though we are pushing against the very grain of our children, and testing society's civility and tolerance at the same time, just for laughs. These expressions mask a whole host of assumptions regarding our rights as sovereign parents with sovereign children. Although these instances are often the exception – their daily, weekly, sometimes monthly occurrence, accumulatively, are enough.

Even in supposedly feminist, pro-women's rights circles, Muslim mothers are denied a legitimate claim to motherhood. As evident in the deafening silence amongst women's rights groups, and indeed the world at large, at the tens of thousands of pregnant women in Gaza, with no healthcare system, many with high risk pregnancies, undergoing the atrocity of caesareans without anaesthesia. While rescuing Muslim mothers from their male counterparts in the name of Western imperialism appears to be a priority for Western foreign policy, the honouring of their agency, life and dignity is not a fashionable or recognised cause outside of this. The Muslim mother exists to flatter Western Imperialism's ego and Western Imperialism's ego alone. We have a very specific purpose in secular ideology, and unless we are participants in our own colonialisation, we are a maligned obstacle in its relentless path.

We know that art is a more effective narrative medium in capturing the hearts and minds of people and yet, as previously mentioned – increasing representation and minority inclusion has been all but redundant in progressing attitudes towards marginalised groups such as Muslims. Some argue that this is the case because in TV, film and drama produced by legacy broadcasters, where the financial incentive is to appeal to majority audiences, the focus of representation rests entirely on individuals, and not communities.

You may be accustomed to seeing a sole Muslim character in your favourite hospital-based serial drama, or soap opera, that is juxtaposed against the standard, default of their white, middle-class backdrop. But Muslim communities remain either entirely absent or vilified – the Muslim in their 'many' is always threatening – for example, the *yawn* terrorist groups, the unruly mob, the clan forcing marriage upon someone etc., etc., ad infinitum... audiences are never exposed to friendly, wholesome Muslim communities, they are only presented with the individual exception to a pretty comprehensively applied dramatic rule.[xxiv]

This echoes with racist sentiments of individuals that will always point at the one black/brown/Muslim friend to exonerate them of their racism, while still squarely attributing harm to their culture and wider communities.[xxv] It also explains the insulting notion of "no-go zones" that is a perennial scare-tactic in Western media – the idea that Muslim majority areas are hostile ghettos for non-Muslims. As a religious culture that places a high value on hospitality and kindness, this is ludicrous to us as Muslims, and exposes the level of projection inherent in racist sentiments; the discomfort of majority society belongs to majority society, minoritised communities should not be deemed responsible for both the cause and effect of irrational bigotry.

The financial incentives behind writing for majority audiences, the lack of diversity behind the camera and in writing rooms, means the impressions created by political and media elite that are pushing their own convenient agenda is not ameliorated by the arts. This goes some way in explaining the almost total dearth of representation of Muslim mothers in particular – even as non-main characters, stalking the very borders of 'community'. And while there are undoubtedly amazing Muslim women in public life who have shattered glass ceiling after glass ceiling and are themselves mothers, very few are presented as mothers in any real public facing way. Perhaps because doing so would detract from the dichotomy we have created between public life and mothering, and 'Muslims' and 'achievement' – it sits in a very uncomfortable conceptual space. The Muslim mother herself, therefore, has no defined public face, when we try to think of one in media, politics and the arts, the mind draws a blank…

So where has motherhood been foregrounded in the court of public opinion for Muslim women and what does it tell us about the impact this symbolic othering and fetishising of Muslim women has on politics and culture, and our everyday lives? One of the most acute expressions of this material reality, which will be more pertinent to younger Muslim mums, is seen in the case of Shamima Begum. Ironically, Begum is framed as the ultimate Muslim Monster according to an increasingly biased media and political commentariat, with her role as a teenage mother during the early days of her media spotlight being integral to the way she was depicted as a national security threat. Shamima, who was heavily pregnant during a series of media interviews when public interest was reignited in February 2019, later tragically went on to lose her child, along with her two previous children.[xxvi] What has since come to light, is that 13-year-old Begum's groomer was in fact a double-agent working for Canadian intelligence,[xxvii] in a textbook case of child grooming and sex trafficking. Not only does her story exemplify how the state – the arbiter of legitimacy – is complicit in creating and cementing the extremism it claims it wants to extinguish, but it also lays bare the tragedy of this for Muslim women – how we are seen as disposable commodities in wider cultural and political wars.

The story sewn by Red Top journalism, intent on towing the Islamophobic line, exemplifies the forged 'othering' narrative and subconscious fears concerning Muslim mothers in full life-cycle, and to its most extreme. Begum was the young girl who, as a Muslim, wasn't afforded a childhood – made culpable for mistakes that international security services baited her into, with the full weight of adult responsibility. Compare this to the debate concerning far-right race rioters of 15 years old, being too young to be prosecuted in 2024, amongst other numerous examples where racialised children are culturally endowed with a sense of responsibility beyond their years.[xxviii] She was the threatening and looming womb – presented as the ultimate danger to Britain. Contrast this with how pregnancy more generally is seen as a time when a woman is at her most vulnerable, and deserving of most sympathy.

And of course she is her mother's daughter – Begum's own mum is continually foregrounded, including in media pieces which defy all journalistic logic; where she has made no comment, yet is centred at the expense of other family members who are actually vocal.[xxix] Of course, this juxtaposes the various instances in which young men racialised as white are depicted as coming from perfect homes and families, in media storms post crime – their criminal acts are portrayed as anomalous to the picture-perfect images that sit neatly under the demurely worded headlines. The blame for Begum's situation in media speak and public imagination appears to be placed with her mother. This echoes the discourse which intensified in the UK under Conservative rule, in which older Muslim mothers were portrayed, condescendingly, in policy terms as both passive victims to their male counterparts, and actively culpable in relation to their children, demonstrating almost perfectly the imagined threat level Muslim mothers supposedly embody.[xxx] Muslim mothers are portrayed as the bridge between one form of Musim criminality and another. It is equally reflective of some of the political instances we see in France – in one an image which reverberated around the world, of a young French Muslim boy sobbing into the shoulder of his veiled mother on a school trip to a regional parliamentary building, as she was labelled a 'provocation' and asked to remove her hijab by a right-wing politician.[xxxi] The Muslim mum is a lightning rod for political actors when they wish to publicly grandstand for their own gain.

Begum herself continues to be stateless to this very day – an explicit threat of the illegitimacy that hangs over Muslim women's heads – and nationally and internationally vilified. The Muslim woman who ultimately followed the state's literal and symbolic desire to be othered and cast beyond their borders, at once British and made unBritish, nationalised and denationalised, veiled and unveiled, mothered and de-mothered, facing a public flogging and sadistically held up as an example, a direct result of their twisted, homespun fantasy. The media exploit Begum's circumstances for front page fodder, fascinated by the woman that is at once everything society reviles and desires in a Muslim woman. Her circumstances and defencelessness remain a twisted triumph for orientalist tropes. Begum's mother herself continues to be portrayed as the sole bearer of responsibility, over and above the state that recruited her daughter, while paradoxically her voice is both symbolised and minimised; amplified and emptied. What she represents is far more important to the world than the reality of her situation.

These facts, of course, reinforce the idea that is pushed upon us, and of course which many of us resist – that as Muslims, we will never really belong in 'The West'. A sentiment that inevitably motivated Begum and her friends to join ISIS, and of course, it is that same sentiment in full action which enabled then Home Secretary, Sajid Javid, to strip her of her citizenship. The irony that those policies which manufactured feelings of disenfranchisement were weaponised against her in dethroning her of her citizenship, is apparently lost on a Government which at the time claimed it enforced counter-terrorism policy in order to protect its own citizens from radicalisation and terror. Maybe deradicalisation policy is aimed squarely at criminalising Muslims, rather than seeking solutions to the security threats the country faces.

The broader context of Begum's situation also exemplifies how Muslim rights are denigrated even epistemically – that is, how our very forms of knowledge and thinking are undermined by a system which devalues religious thinking, and marginalises specifically Muslim truths. This is evident in how scholars, religious leaders and Muslim authorities on Islam are denied when they condemn barbaric acts that are ostensibly carried out in the name of Islam. Compare this to how Christian leaders' thoughts and statements are given legitimacy and weight when they denounce extreme acts carried out in the name of Christianity. Secular, Islamophobic culture is so self-centredly arrogant it purports to know more about Islam than us as Muslims – it claims the intellectual upper hand, placing themselves as experts, even when it comes to our own faith. This belittling of Muslim thinking is also evident in those instances where Muslim mothers are treated with condescension concerning the decisions they make for their own children, there is this infantilising treatment we receive as adults making informed decisions about our own lives and values.

The case of Shamima Begum remains an abject symbol of gendered Islamophobia and what that means for Muslim women in all of its brute, crude and tragic fashion. Her experience simultaneously projects the nation's worst fears regarding the looming security threat of the Muslim youth, and many of our own fears as Muslim women, concerning our sense of belonging and rootedness. Her case captures that strange no man's land of identity that many of us feel we exist in, between a deafening political climate which constantly renders us as other, and our own precarious sense of belonging in, in this case, British culture. The media's caricature of Begum and her current statelessness is an explicit depiction of the threat that exists for Muslim women the country over. The irony that a falsified 'extreme' Islam was used to both draw her into one end of the secular fantasy – 'jihadi bride' – and that it was a self-identified Muslim Home Secretary that cast her in the role of the opposite fetish – as stateless nomad – by revoking her citizenship. Two sides of a worryingly similar coin.

If we want to make a trivial parable of what remains a profoundly depressing situation, Begum is British Islamophobia's own unique Frankenstein – an identity forged by normative social attitudes, a hostile political climate, and regressive and punitive policies.

How we perceive ourselves as Muslim Mothers

The underlying issues that came to light from Begum and her mothers' case embodies many of the binary contradictions upon which many Muslim mothers' identities are based, and how we ourselves internalise it in unproductive and damaging ways. The media held up images of the woman too Muslim to be deemed British when she was veiled in a refugee camp with her then living child, and then too 'Westernised' to fit populist notions of Muslimness as a de-veiled young Muslim woman; though none of them earned her humanisation. The dichotomy it supposedly upholds is that we must be one or the other – Western, deserving of humanity, or Muslim and deserving of none. Begum was brought up with this dichotomy, and yet to the media, it is her Muslimness that her crimes are attributed to, and not her Britishness. In the same way this same media are always ready to claim Muslim/minoritised sports stars as British, American or French when they score the winning goal. How that part of their identity is posited as the site of potential good, and it is the Muslim part of their identity that is ready to absorb deviance and in need to temperance. As though we are only half worthy, and that half only when it is exceptional.

Often times, it is the things that are unspoken that have so much power. It is the insidious nature of these stereotypes that cause the most damage to us. That this process of Otherisation remains largely unnamed and unknown, existing only on the below-surface level of headlines and cinematic plots which seek to dehumanise, is perhaps its most damaging feature. It is a kind of enthymeme – a falsehood not stated directly, but assumed by a cultural narrative that tacitly reinforces this falsehood as an underlying premise. In this way, the cultural fiction that we as Muslims are aberration is presumed, part of that underside on which secular existence sits, and so enters our mind with a silent validation, an unchallenged presupposition – it is therefore much harder to guard against.

This goes hand in hand with the idea that Muslim hate is quite literally undefinable, and in politics today we are still debating what linguistic shape Islamophobia takes. The reticence of the political classes in applying legal definitions also suggests they attribute – or dog whistle – a kind of legitimacy to anti-Muslim prejudice, suggesting it is a natural and accepted kind of intellectual disposition. The unspoken nature of this kind of bigotry is also a convenient tool which allows an implicit and tacit calling to anti-Muslim hate, without those instigating it ever having to be called up on its consequences. There is no barometer by which to hold those who shape public conversation in this way, accountable – Islamophobia is a hateful scripture which leaves no discernible fingerprints or residue for those that wish to advance it.

As Muslims, this tacit culture means we don't possess the everyday language to define this broader phenomenon, and therefore combat it ourselves. The idea that we exist on a spectrum of Muslimness to Humanness, and that each move in one direction compromises our position on the other, has become part of our unconscious training. It's a reflection of the shape-shifting nature of the conceptual Muslim, which we've discussed and which remains an amorphous figure, ready to adapt to the profile of the next social angst.

This inevitably impacts us personally as Muslim mums who are navigating through, and bringing up our children against this ideological backdrop. How we internalise our Islam is perhaps the most critical thing when we are initial torch bearers for that Islam amongst our own children.

We have absorbed on a molecular, non-verbal level, this binary that has come to define the world around us. We will always fall into the habit of justifying our existence and practices, and define ourselves either by or against this construct of The Muslim. We will feel an inclination to distance ourselves from symbols of Muslimness that we deem 'too' Muslim, and beliefs and practices that are not repackaged in liberal terminology. We often struggle to express Islam, as it is, a beautiful balance of faith and doctrine – prescribed actions rooted in a love and submission to God. Religion is deemed acceptable according to secular and Western constructs when it is either 'exotic' and 'mystically' nebulous, or deemed unrigid and flexible, like a liberating shamanism. Islam fits neither of these categories because it's not subject to man-made desires, its belief and practice requires a necessary humility, and it is Divinely constructed, beyond our capabilities and sometimes our immediate understanding too.

To do anything for the sake of God, or for a higher purpose that doesn't revel in the shallowness of the surface of the self, creates a reflexive, knee-jerk repulsion, and the strength and unconscious nature of this impulse alone is telling. There appears to be something deeply superstitious, parochial and "backward" about Islamic faith that is part of our very instinctive perception of it. And this exhibits itself in Muslim women, and mothers, in varying ways. And naturally, this will have a domino effect on how our children perceive and express their faith.

To some extent, we are at risk of seeing ourselves as this very shape-shifting, nefarious Muslim. What is *halal* and wholesome in Islam becomes a kind of "*haram*" according to wider society that has the potential to cause a kind of cognitive dissonance and self-aberration in us as Muslims. It seems we are forced into a corner of either embracing this ugly caricature of the Muslim, or denouncing Islam entirely. In regards to the former, abhorrent terror groups, with no claim to Islam, such as ISIS, feed off of the warped perception we have of our own selves. If the Muslim comes to be everything that isn't rational, speakable, humanistic, then the more irrational, inhumane, unspeakable something becomes is a marker of how 'Muslim' we see it. We have effectively created a positive correlation between 'Muslimness' and barbarism, that ISIS's own savagery plays neatly into, and that has us tacitly affirming Islamic practice on perverse bases. ISIS employ this binary, and exploit this unspoken affiliation in us, as a marketing tool. The more 'anti-Western' they project themselves, the more it taps into a falsely constructed idea within us of what is legitimately Muslim. They have identified the negative space of ideological meaning that many of us are at risk of defining our faith by. And this is the reason that Muslims erroneously joined ISIS when it formed, and remains one of the reasons we as a community need to be vigilant about what migrates into our perception of faith.

One stark illustration of this phenomenon is Begum's own account of joining ISIS – 'I wanted to be a good Muslim' she told media outlets in 2021.[xxxii] How woefully tragic and utterly depressing that a young girl saw what ISIS represents as the ultimate expression of Islam. This measure of Muslimness as the ultimate symbol of bruteness, and how it impresses upon our finer instincts, means that the greatest victim of Islamophobia is ultimately our faith.

[Director's notes: What goes without saying, of course, but bears mentioning here, is that Islam is not restricted to one end of the globe and many of the Muslims throughout the world – prime amongst them myself – do wholly inhabit their Western and Muslim identities. Homogenising everything 'Eastern' as Muslim has its own very scary pitfalls which we will go on to probe in the next chapter, in the same way that reducing everything 'Western' to anti-Muslim is fundamentally flawed. Islam is a conscious endeavour, which requires an active effort from all of us, not a lazy descension into culture or customary norms. Despite attempts to racialise Islam, and reduce it to an ethnology, it remains resolutely a theology open to all, irrespective of cultural affiliation or background. We can and will love the Western culture we belong to, and see no contradiction in embodying both. And of course, Islamophobia itself originated from the Middle East, it's very fathers are Bani Qureish – a fact that disrupts the simplistic binary we have outlined, and which will certainly hurt many Islamophobes desperate to invent ethnopurity, when it very rarely exists. The fact is that both what represents itself as "Islamism" and "secularism" are two sides of the same coin, that seek to pervert our faith into the same twisted caricature.]

And so, as Muslim mothers living in a globalised culture of Islamophobia, many of us have internalised Islam and Muslim identity as a deficit model; something defined in opposition to secular liberalism, a restrictive force if you like, holding us back from the default standard of a liberal lifestyle. Muslims are NOT allowed to… [add an endless list of verbs here]. The idea that Islam is a stand-alone system in and of itself is something we have to consciously bring into our thought space – the fact that it is also nourishing, fulfilling, bringing infinite value, is something we have to train ourselves to understand. For those rooted in mainstream culture, the draw to perceive, and sometimes even enact, practices as large as abstinence from alcohol, and as small as eating with your right hand, as though it is the opposite of the default way of doing something, rather than affirmatively as part of a divine system which exists in its own right, is strong

It is the othering of us that impacts our self-impression, that as Mums we must be cognisant of. Young Muslim women who are living in an age of information, with digital tools at their disposal, are in a better position than ever to empower themselves with the knowledge, learning, and unlearning to combat much of what we have navigated. As we explored previously – as media and information systems become more democratised, and we are now on the verge of developing a truly plural landscape of political narratives, for the first time ever, we may see a generation that grows up without the hang-ups and stigmatisation concerning their faith. Coupled with the slow death of legacy media and the impact of the economic models and financial incentives of streaming services – which require a diverse range of subscribers, rather than mainstream or majority appeal – we are likely to see more varied voices in the creative industries, and therefore more wholesome and accurate representation on our screens.[xxxiii] The cultural atmosphere within which we mother, and which our children are raised, is on the verge of significant changes, and it is a poignant time for mothers of our generation who are also amongst the most well-informed and most active in undoing some of those intergenerational harms that we have identified in this epoch of Muslim mothering, *al-ḥamdulillāh*.[21]

As possessors of truth, we have the greatest resource at hand to help weed out our internal biases concerning ourselves. In the same way we need to unpick our self-image from the thorny intrusion of the male gaze, from social expectations as a tribe of women; as political beings, we also need to unpick it from the piercing forces of Islamophobia.

---

[21] All Praise to Allāh

How we parent as Muslim Other

As discussed, and as we will go onto dissect in more detail, many of the issues we face as Muslim mums are also structural. Because of this, we often experience the weight of racism in our interface with public institutions, and this spans almost uniformly from the cradle to the grave. Take for example maternity services on both sides of the Atlantic, and the poor experience Muslim women – overwhelmingly from racialised communities in Western contexts – are often subject to, and which translates into racial stereotyping about pain tolerance, microaggressions, and, most tragically, stark racial disparities in maternal mortality rates.[xxxiv,xxxv,xxxvi] Carry this through to the way some elderly Muslim women are treated, again, by health services, and the 'Mrs Bibi' syndrome affecting often Muslim, South Asian women presumed to be exaggerating their health concerns.[xxxvii]

As parents our most acute concerns regarding these institutional biases will centre on our children, and will naturally impact the very way we mother – these are the very institutions through which we navigate life; the educational settings our children spend the majority of their formative years, the health institutions we turn to when we are in need and the security and legal institutions we fall on when we are often at our most vulnerable. In Western countries a deep suspicion of Muslims is written into these institutional structures through anti-terror ideology. Anti-terror ideology is the meeting place of all those fluid and crystalised notions of Muslim as threat, danger, opposite to 'normal'. It's the legal, social and cultural expression of all those anxieties in full force. It is the key to much of how Muslim society is vilified and therefore impairs our sense of faith and our ability, and will, to parent as Muslim mothers. Though theorists and policy makers are at pain to say they are separate, there is a convergence in how violent extremism and non-violent extremism is perceived and tackled globally, and what this means for how our faith is implicated in an environment where it is deemed aberrant.[xxxviii]

This much, and more, is evident in the neologism 'Islamism' which is what's most often used, globally, to describe supposedly Muslim terror activity and which represents the closing of a conceptual and rhetorical gap, and the ultimate converging of 'Muslim' and 'Monster' as identities. This migration of rhetorical terms from innocuous to legally and criminally binding, via social and cultural use and perception, is also evident in how 'Allāh*u*

Akbar[22] appears to be going through an evolutionary process in public and media imagination. We have now reached the Overton Window – the process by which previously unacceptable notions become acceptable through public reference – where it may be deemed a criminal term, with one British Member of Parliament suggesting uttering the term is an arrest-worthy offence.[xxxix]

These instances demonstrate how the very concept of our faith is colonised through those words we use to conceive of and express it. How the building blocks of what makes up our very expression of faith are twisted and distorted for the benefit of domestic politics and the military industrial complex. The attempt to colonise the very tongue and ideology concerning Islam is now foraying into our own private worship too, with these repeated attempts to illegalise, tarnish, and interdict expressions of worship as "controversial" due to "associations with extremism" by mainstream British Media.[xl] These bad faith actions only serve to pathologise Islam and add to the blanket of securitisation we face as Muslim communities. For Muslims, in how we mother, this presents an array of issues.

---

[22] God is Great

Much of the particularly British, French and American perceptions of this realm of policy and practice are presupposed on the idea of the widely debunked 'conveyor belt' model which creates a positive correlation between religiously conservative views and potential for radicalisation. For Muslims in many Western contexts, religiosity becomes a possible indicator of vulnerability to radicalisation – for example under a non-violent extremism logic, developing an interest in prayer and refraining from celebrating other religious festivals become red flags for potentially violent extremist thought and behaviour. This carves out a dangerous and nebulous 'pre-crime' space in the British legal system in particular, muddying the already muddled legal and social understanding of Muslims. It is both speculative and highly intrusive of Muslims, particularly children and young people, and emboldens those with a duty of care to Muslim children to act upon racist hunches. Due to the white noise of Islamophobia in the UK, much of what we deem suspicious is Islamic faith, and what we deem as Islamic faith is suspicious, leading to Muslim children being overwhelmingly referred to an unnerving system and programme without even coming remotely near the threshold of 'terror' or 'threat to the state'.[xli]

In the context of the UK, this has created a very culture in itself – a 'Prevent' culture, which is welded together through the various strands of anti-terror policy, strategy and guidance. The Prevent strategy in the UK, which puts a statutory duty on public service professionals to report *potential* signs of radicalisation, views Muslim practice through the lens of suspicion, and deems Islamic thought a threat to domestic security. Prevent, and the British approach in particular, is widely lauded by national and international terror experts for achieving the opposite to its stated aims by creating disenfranchisement amongst the Muslim population, and creating cultural tensions and divisions.[xlii] It's often referred to as policy informed evidence, rather than evidence informed policy due to its ineffective review and implementation.[xliii] It is effectively racist assumptions enshrined in law, and is arrogantly self-referential.

Ultimately, it drives expressions of Muslimness underground as illicit, further convoluting and polluting our impressions of our faith. As mentioned, it questions the very legitimacy of Muslim belief, and our credibility as parents with supposedly full rights, as a result. Due to the illegitimacy that counter-terror thinking presumes on Islam and Muslim parenting, and because Islam and Muslims are infantilised due to an abstinence and stoicism that omits certain activities seen as akin to 'adulthood', Islam is perceived as a transitionary and potentially volatile phase, something we need to move on from and grow out of. It is the state's job, of course, to police this growth and spiritual maturity, as though they are hurrying us along from loitering in the corridor towards humanity. And as with all these damaging tropes, it is entirely reflected in how we ourselves perceive our faith, and particularly what are deemed more 'orthodox' elements of it. As Muslims living in a globalised age, we often see religious practice and thinking as a short-lived trend, that those periods we are more wed to our faith are actually a kind of immaturity, a stumbling back into delusion before we allow the 'real world' to set in and awake us from this unproductive stupor.

Much of this tension created by counter-terror policy and Muslims lies in domestic-adjacent spaces such as the school.

Just like the family and home become the projected sites of social anxiety, schools as buffers between the domestic and state spheres are subject to a similar level of hysteria in policy making. What greater foothold does the state have into the home than through the education of children. And built into this education system is all manner of entitlements and assumptions about norms and defaults in morality. The panic over Muslim homes and British families was always going to have the most virulent expression in education policy. And this is not to mention the colonial hang-ups concerning education as a civilising force. We have seen this in recent prayer bans at high profile schools[xliv] and of course the Trojan Horse Scandal – one of the most obtrusive events on the landscape of British policy making for Muslims, and which led to the real-time crystallisation of institutional Islamophobia.[xlv]

This assumption that Muslim children, as potential receptacles of terror, might need to be safeguarded from their parents, purely by virtue of their faith is what underpins Prevent culture in public institutions.[xlvi] The fundamentalist view that, primarily, a child is by nature secular (again that any forms of parenting, and children's development more generally can be deemed 'natural' is what is truly telling) moreover, that the Islamic belief system is unnatural to that child, and that they are otherwise intended on a liberal life-path, reveals the regressive attitudes towards Muslims and Islam, and the cultural blind spots that policy makers on the highest level possess.

The case studies relating to Prevent referrals are themselves very worrying – with many parents citing it as a traumatic event for their child. The insidious nature of anti-Muslim sentiment means that Muslim children are not always afforded the same childhood as some of their non-racialised counterparts. The reality for Muslim children is that misspelt words, haphazard drawings, misheard statements and absolutely normal childhood behaviour can result in referrals to police, interviews and records on the government's counter-terror policing database for six years. Criminalisation by any other name. The contemporary notion of childhood, with its roots in a Victorian Britain with evolving social constructs, isn't conceptually large enough to accommodate children of Muslim heritage. Freedom, creativity and innocence isn't as easily attributed to them, and dangerous presumptions, and surveying institutional eyes, follow them on the basis of their religious heritage alone.

As a parent, internalising the Islamophobic gaze is often part of that protective measure you must assume as a parent to safeguard your child from the trauma of this frankly mad, yet entirely plausible, chain of events. The paradoxical position of having to be cognisant of your child's behaviour through the hateful lens of Islamophobic legislation is in itself a fraught experience, and that's without the anxiety of all of its consequences. When Muslim parents are in any kind of health or educational setting it causes a hypervigilance and self-othering that is unnerving and counterproductive to true social cohesion, and which imbues dangerous cadences onto our impressions of our faith. This is of course worse for some Muslim mothers than others – for example black Muslim mothers who have to bear double the weight due to the perverse criminalisation of black children and young people in particular. It leaves many of us as mothers contemplating a kind of micro-dosing of Islamophobia to our children to prepare them for the onslaught they will be witness to in their adult life. Wondering how much harm to expose them to, to limit further harm – a very unnerving weighing up of how much to wake them from the sweet stupor of childhood innocence before someone else does it with the crushing blow of such an ugly reality.

For many parents in the UK, and other countries with legislature and guidance that effectively criminalises Muslim faith, these policy positions signal a blithe disregard for their children. There is something ludicrous about these small, navel-gazing governments attempting to delegitimise a legitimate global religion that exposes them as both small-minded and parochial in approach. It means as Muslim mothers, we have to be bigger, expand ourselves to absorb the shocks inherent in a state that often neglects our children, and to square up to the overbearing ideology that renders them wrong. It means we have to assume an additional layer of protectiveness and impermeability so we are able to guard our children from some of those intrusions.

Due to how guarded the Prevent guidance is, case studies are necessary to allow us to connect some of the dots concerning this heavily shrouded approach – one that data evidences leads to a high number of false referrals of Muslims.[xlvii] Accumulatively, it demonstrates how each racist assumption, every ill-informed judgement and every ignorant prejudice is encouraged to sediment and erect an ugly edifice of racism that upholds many public structures including in health and education. They also make apparent the perverse logic and paradoxical nature of anti-terror wisdom. Often ill-informed individuals are able to testify against Muslim children and families, simply referencing their mere 'belief' that those families are a threat. The state in its very apparatus, encourages and supports these individual's beliefs concerning the threat these Muslim families pose to the UK, while undermining the same religious beliefs of those identified; mostly innocuous observances such as private prayer and abstaining from certain celebrations outside of Islam, as previously mentioned. The cannibalistic nature of anti-terror thinking is woefully apparent here – seemingly not all beliefs are created equal. It also exposes the weak foundations of institutional Islamophobia – as whimsical, arbitrary and completely lacking in substance or truth. And all this, in true counter-terror logic, to protect the threatening and vulnerable Muslim child. This conflating of Muslim with danger means, in practice, professionals with safeguarding duties to Muslim children must assume the role of securing the nation from potential (Muslim-child-shaped) terror, and often under the guise of child protection, those children will be referred to state security professionals for their own supposed safeguarding. A kind of inversion that really exemplifies the clarity, direction and purpose of such laws and guidance.

Furthermore, what is also implicit in the Prevent narrative is the idea that religious or Islamic thought comes at the expense of children's safety, success or cultural enrichment. The irony of claiming Islam is culturally deficient, while holding the most reductionist view of Islam oneself, is not lost on many of us. Prevent further stigmatises and alienates Muslim children in the name of assimilating them into British life, stifling their true development socially, culturally, academically and professionally.

Through Prevent, and its enactment, the Muslim is projected as clandestine, lacking cultural scope and academic ambition, ignorant, nihilistic, and destructive towards other cultures and people, using women and children as tools to further their own ideological agenda. Indeed, the fingerprints left on the Muslim community show us that the political elite have sculpted the perfect image of themselves in their fiction. What Prevent makes most apparent is perhaps the danger doesn't lie within Muslim communities.

The "soft" impact of this is of course how we parent culturally amidst this political climate and how that impacts customs and norms we bring into our home. Muslim mums will feel a subliminal resistance in how we embody, practice, and teach our faith. As though it is a secret language we must censor in front of others, like a subterranean, behind-closed-doors ideology that shouldn't see the oxygen of public life. The infamous getting caught with your foot in the sink, or the *athan*[23] alarm going off on the bus of modern

---

23 Call to prayer

internet lore really exemplifies our subconscious thoughts regarding the "public" facing nature of what we consider our "private faith". Ironically, Islam is one of the few faiths that defines itself as a way of life – there is no English equivalent to the Arabic term *din* – the closest translation to 'faith'. A fact which exemplifies how beautifully whole, total and fulfilling it is – how much of it is inherently incorruptible and rooted in our relationship with our Creator. And yet because of social, political and cultural standards, we have been pressured to reduce our faith so it is the most passive, compartmentalised, silent and hidden.

There is a perennial sense of illegitimacy attributed to Islam that means we will strive towards the illusive quality of being an acceptable level of secular. As parents with an instinctive bond with our children, there is absolutely no doubt that they will inherit, on some level, this sense of clandestine and illicitness that we have effectively ascribed to our faith. It is that worming feeling when your child says 'Allāh*u Akbar*' in the queue at the supermarket– the hesitation when your daughter says she wants to wear hijab to the park. The 'what will they say' Muslim-edit, that makes us second guess every faith act and expression and which exposes the shortfall we deem between our beliefs and practices and what's perceived as acceptable and proper enough for public consumption. It is that invisible noose around our necks that closes in on our very expression of faith. It may programme you to second guess your decisions concerning what values you affirm as a family, what expression this forms in terms of commemorating or celebrating festivals, wearing outward symbols of faith, conforming to visible practices – there seems to always be some bargaining concerning our expression of faith that invites the invisible eye of public scrutiny and the popular gaze into that intimate space where our actions and motivations as Muslims resides. As Muslims we can sometimes end up parenting on auto-pilot – conforming to secular practices with a kind of forced enthusiasm that is itself telling. That speaks so much of all the internal training we've received, from our own formative years, of what we deem we must do to be perceived – by ourselves and others – as human or worthy. It also speaks of how much we are at risk of passing that on to the next generation of Muslims, and the intergenerational impact of Islamophobia (To finish the job that Disney's *Aladdin* so crudely began…).

This creates a kind of social toxicity that makes every parental decision for Muslims in the West a minefield in which we must balance our child's spiritual and social welfare, the weight of social expectations and the looming, long arm of the law. The mental tax on Muslim mothers as a result can be great. As Muslim children age, these values come into sharper contrast, with often natural conflicts between parent and child concerning changing values, peer pressure and other external factors having the potential to carry a greater weight due to this perceived criminalisation, and apparently illegitimate nature of perfectly harmless beliefs and practices. The state effectively sanctions a narrative that Islam is the 'wrong' way to parent. The idea that we as Muslim mums are standing resolutely, often sinisterly, in the way of the apparently organic tide of liberalism is one that takes on different internal and external tensions in different stages of our parenting, and adds unnecessary friction to the connections we have with our children.

This is before we broach the subject of aspirations – what we as Muslim mothers want for our children in material terms. The very idea of being upwardly mobile, or aspirational, centres on bourgeoise notions of middle class culture. Middle class culture, particularly within French and British models of social classification, is inherently racialised, and particularly exclusionary of Muslim culture – as we've touched on previously.

When we deconstruct different barometers for success within British society, for example, this becomes patently obvious. If we are defining middle class aspirations in educational terms (and in Britain, where educational attainment of the child is linked specifically to their parents' level of education, not wealth, or other determiners, this is a pertinent benchmark) then perhaps we should ask ourselves why West African migrants to the UK, overwhelmingly of degree level qualification or higher, are not deemed 'middle class' in the British context? If we pivot slightly and instead use the endeavour to achieve, and a valuing of educational achievement as our definition of middle class, then why do Bengali families who are taking greater strides in education, by day, not fit into our conception of middle class families? If we go bohemian, and use cultural capital and affinity towards arts and culture as a marker of middle class communities – then can't we say British Somalis, who are immersed in a rich heritage of poetry, fit into that bracket? And if we use good old cash, money, and even a little bit of bling, as our primary measure, then surely wealthy entrepreneurial Pakistani's in towns such as Luton or Birmingham, who dominate many of the local private schools are themselves middle class? The answer of course is that in most people's imagination these are not, and cannot be middle class communities. Rather, Muslims are deemed inherently uncouth, and only considered middle class or aspirational if they assume what are construed as white or secular characteristics.

As Muslim mothers, we need to radically redefine who and what we deem as aspirational for our children, on our own terms and outside this narrow thinking. This includes our own cultural biases concerning what we perceive as aspirational educational trajectories – where we can see the Muslim world is dominated by brilliant minds in STEM, we have a dearth of great minds in media or the arts, where this imbalance is felt so acutely on a cultural level. A common trend amongst some Muslim families is to deny their children access to any classical arts, history and other culture because it is seen as superfluous, irrelevant or because we are intimidated by it. This creates a generation of Muslims who are at risk of being culturally blindsided – unable to navigate the realities of the world they inhabit, visually, historically or politically – think of how a lack of visual literacy has led to the denigration of specifically Muslim women that we outlined previously, or more pertinently how we are unable to take from the lessons of history to make sense of our political present. This thinking also denies our children any creative, *halal* outlet, ironically amongst a backdrop where we are vocally obsessive about avoiding *haram*. Very often, Muslim families will feel channelling any energy in these endeavours is wasteful, leaving those teens with no other recreational purpose than to scroll through their phones, wasting a kind of creative and cultural potential that is fertile ground for a healthy sense of self-esteem and purpose. While it is naturally unproductive to unquestioningly revere art, or put all historical figures on a pedestal – the movements for decolonisation, and our faith itself makes this much obvious – it is equally reactionary and counterproductive to dismiss the creative realm entirely as many of us do.

Living beyond binaries

I am willing to state, almost unequivocally, that the one thing that unites us as we shroud around this book, and cast our eyes over these very words, is that our utmost priority is our child's faith. Despite the many backgrounds, cultures, life paths we have taken to get to this very point, we are bound by this unending and irrepressible desire to give our children what we believe is the best quality known to man – the beauty of submission to Him. And this maternal instinct is itself telling because many of us might be trained to qualify this drive with caveats such as '..and be a good person..' or any other number of platitudes. But the fact remains, on some non-verbal level we understand that to be a Muslim *is* to incorporate all of those, what we may consider, liberal-adjacent notions of moral goodness. For our children to be Muslim *is* for our children to be good, decent, hard-working, high achieving, socially-conscious, civic, environmentally conscious... and the list is endless. All qualities we are told our religion isn't, and which are themselves natural consequences of our worship of Allāh. To follow the noble tradition of our Prophet ﷺ is the apex of that standard of humanity we begin to deconstruct and revaluate when we become mothers – and the inverse is true too; to be the best is to emulate our Prophet ﷺ. And that's because despite the layers of social construction, those extrinsic pressures, Allāh has blessed us with an intrinsic kernel of truth from which our *imaan* blossoms, and which we need to cultivate through *taqwā*.[24] What distinguishes us from the world, and unites us as Muslim mums, is that we understand that our children need Islam in the very bones that hold us up – we are intimately aware, as bringers of life, that this life needs to worship Allāh.

---

[24] God consciousness

Indeed, the very fact that we stand here as Muslim mums, despite the unique challenges that are sometimes thrown our way as a result, is a testament to His truth. It's a testament to His Mercy. The only humanly intelligible parable which Allāh cites for this, is the mother herself. The role Allāh has assigned us as mothers and mere creation, is to help to inculcate this beauty of our submission, through the mercy He's imbued us with as a total blessing.

The problem with binaries is they shoehorn our thinking. We begin to either see ourselves as The Muslim Other, or the opposite to The Muslim Other, amongst which true Islam is lost. And it is the fact that we often absorb deficient notions of a system we define ourselves by, and which we willingly ascribe to. This leads to a kind of internalised contradiction that we need to be cognisant of. It means we can adopt Islam as though it is merely a senseless tradition. The off shoot of this has led to a silent phenomenon in which we overwhelmingly parent from fear – assuming our children won't value the immaterial, transcendental reinforcement of Islam. We project our own unconscious assumptions onto our children and fall into an autopilot of parenting that lacks meaning, definition and purpose.

The feeling of fear, and unconscious parenting, comes from this poverty of understanding – and often this deficit model upon which we base our impressions of Islam – our impression of Islam comes from the position we inhabit, living in the margins of society. Without taking hold of our faith, and redrafting our impression of it, it becomes an admission of our own spiritual and religious impoverishment, of our inability to value those intangible benefits that come with our religion. The climate of Islamophobia is in danger of immiserating our faith if left unhindered. If we don't consciously value something, how can we attribute a worth to it in our homes, and set that precedent as parents. For some of us this fear may be because we accepted Islam from a foreign tongue, or even a culture that was alien to us, so we imagine our children's impression of Islam will be the same as our own – lacking definition, meaning and purpose. All of us, born Muslim or not, came to a point where we consciously chose Islam for ourselves. A moment where we understood that we were holding this baton of Islam in the wider race of life. And that spiritual tussle, that realisation, awareness and understanding, is so intimately personal. It is rooted in the very crevices of our consciousness. As parents that are tasked with extending it forward, it is an intricate and often clouded process, but one that offers such hope and beauty.

The idea that is socially constructed around us, that Islam in its purest form is the most monstrous and brutish of things, has coloured our language and crucially our thinking, in so many ways – it has us introducing qualifying terms such as 'moderate' or 'extreme' Muslim to our lexicon. To overcome this descent into the linguistically nebulous, and increasing encroachment on our faith, is of course to give our religion shape and meaning on terms rooted in Islamic scholarship, and not secular myths and fallacies. To give Islam the oxygen of language – fill this gaping rhetorical space – and to air it from the bind it's been held in at the benefit of opposing identities starts with piecing that language and value system together, through learning Islam, interrogating our presumptions, making the Quran our companion and His religion our supreme guide. If we define ourselves by the very language we speak, then as English-speaking Muslims perhaps it is time we adopt a new way of speaking and perceiving of our faith.

While so much is written and spoken about regarding not bringing unwanted baggage to parenting, less is said about the cultural and secular baggage concerning Islam that we carry with us into the role of motherhood. Minimal, if any, light is shone on how much work we need to do to unpack our feelings around faith, to understand that the wider bubble of hate is a debate that secular liberalism is having with itself. We need only to disentangle our religious heritage, and stop allowing our identity, belief and practice to be dependent upon and intimately tied to others.

As we've examined, secular notions of progress are linear, with Enlightenment as the apex of human development. That is, modern anthropology tells us that monotheism was bred from tribes refining themselves into nation states, and with that, man worshipping multiple gods to the refinement and concept of a single god. It tells us that the trajectory of humanity reached its final and most edifying destination by celebrating human intellect alone and it is the self that is great.

Conversely, the Quran teaches us that Islam is the destination, and height, of progress – man was blessed with fitrah and deviated, only to be reminded of the Oneness of Allāh by successive Prophets. Our religious idea of progress does not follow this linear model which places the birth of the nuclear bomb and warfare as its crowning jewel.

Our meta-narrative teaches that there is something greater than us – Allāh. And that we understand this through humility to Him and not aggrandisement of the self. In fact, it teaches us that human intellect is fallible, and gives us the tools to overcome complacency and not engender it. It teaches us that we can make mistakes without damning ourselves – indeed to sin and have the humility to truly repent is far greater than not sinning at all; emphasising the importance placed in Islam on endeavour, of that sense of striving. We need to actively confront and tackle our inadequacies rather than wallow in the self-indulgence of hubris and distraction. Islam reminds us that these weaknesses are opportunities for strength, *inshā'Allāh* [25] and that not all social influence is good, and certainly not all of it is bad. It teaches us nuance, the quest for continual self-progression and dignity. All values that secular, liberal ideology is labouring to achieve. And while our default position as social animals when it comes to discerning meaning and value is to fall back lazily on binaries, Islam encourages a more reflective, conscious and active means by which to understand and shape the world.

---

[25] God willing

While humanity has been debating the duality of the body and mind – Christianity traditionally denigrating its demands and late-stage capitalism celebrating and centring unadulterated its pleasures, Islam teaches us that the perfect practice exists when we engage both – an act gains *barakat* through both intention of the mind and practice of the limbs. This means we need to be conscious of how we allow other false binaries to root themselves in our thinking and practice. And this will undoubtably cause discomfort, but those of us that remain in the domain of absolute comfort are rarely given the opportunity to grow. That sphere of disquiet is often where we find the grit and integrity to be better.

Perhaps, as mothers and believers, it is time for us to relearn and reclaim our identity on more nuanced, honest and self-reflective terms. To question those unthinking, impulsive urges. To confront our weaknesses rather than distract from them. To look beyond ourselves, to a greater and wider narrative, but certainly not for the purpose of unquestioningly affirming oneself. To be humble. And off the back of all this, maybe tell secular humanism a story or two.

CHAPTER 4

THE CULTURAL: PROPAGENDER AND CULTURING THE MUSLIM MOTHER

"And we have created you in pairs." (An-Naba 78:8)

There are close to a million pixels on the average phone screen. A million pixels which mediate our reality – through which we blend and assimilate our world and the place we occupy within it. These millions of information carrying, light harbouring, minute cells act as vacuums into an asymmetrical, almost parasitic realm that shapes more and more of the modern world. Through the phones that inveigled themselves into the minutiae of our lives, our laptop screens, and other digital devices, we are shaping and feeding our physical, ideological and cultural appetites. We order our evenings take away through delivery apps, with a side of gender ideology via YouTube shorts, we book the weekends' gallery visit just after a left swipe from an incoherent rant on migrants, made by a sorry soul calling in to the local radio show. In return for this attention bondage, we deposit a digital fingerprint which is used to further bind us into this increasingly exploitative relationship. Our natural instincts of consumption are dissected, digitised, plotted and analysed so they can be distilled, purified and honed to perpetuate that consumption ad infinitum. The highly processed foods we are inviting into our bodies mirror the highly processed information systems by which we are forming our deepest held beliefs and values, and living our lives. These unassuming little pixels that we give credence to and elevate to the status of cultural foremen, have wielded seismic change in the real world – they have fomented the kind of culture wars that have forged new frontiers in the ideological order, synthesising different values and beliefs and which have therefore welded together new norms from the tatters of what existed before them.

Often times what passes for cultural 'progress' in the online world is really a regressive lie sold to us as novelty. For example, the internet's perennial obsession with the 1950s as an idealised time for wages, living standards, and most pertinently, gender ideals. The 50s is rhapsodised by proponents of this idealism and modern lore as a reflection of a more natural gender equilibrium – the way we are all *supposed* to be. In reality, it is no coincidence that this period marked the advent of capitalism and the synthesis of consumer culture, and what we understand of it is actually a twee, cutesy reimagining of it by mercenary film and TV industries. This inherent contradiction reverberates through the idealisms it propagates, as we will go on to interrogate.

But nowhere is the relationship between man and internet more exploitative, more David-and-Goliath, than when it comes to the woman and female interests at large. The internet is based upon a binary code which further dichotomises and polarises the world it impresses upon. While it continues to create rapid changes in our cultural topography – dating etiquettes, gender definitions and racial attitudes are all examples of where the internet has created such drastic ripples – it also has a simultaneously reversing impact by cementing certain bigotries that are intrinsic to the ecosystem as a whole.

The more 'progressive' the trends we see on the internet, the more extreme the 'opposite' of these trends will come to emerge, as a natural consequence of how the internet is structured and how it shapes our existence. This binary nature of the internet, and the divisive social architecture it creates, means the contrived male vs. female dynamic was always the most vulnerable to manipulation on digital terrain, and that women are more often disadvantaged by it. Gender divisions are exacerbated by online discourse, disinformation and posturing, and women face further adversity as a result. With rising cases of femicide, anti-female hate is increasingly being seen as a form of terrorism by governments rushing to keep up with the ripples created by online movements. Likewise, the age old trope of Muslim as 'other', the rabbit hole from which we have just come up for air, provides the perfect blueprint for a divisive internet culture to so neatly map itself upon. Muslims face more hostility both in and because of online dynamics. This means, the Muslim online world, and the Muslim, female online world are both key cell-cultures in the social laboratory of the internet, and this is critical to the culture we absorb and propagate as Muslim mothers. While we may not think that internet cultures – niche, underground or mainstream – impact the everyday Muslim's ideals, values and intellectual capacity, the opposite is true. Some of the subcultures we will navigate in this chapter go from esoteric and specialist, to mainstream and every day; crossing the cultural barrier into the ubiquity of playground rhymes and every day vernacular, with lightning speed. What happens online very rarely stays online, and some digital cultures, habits and attitudes act as a bellwether, giving us an insight into future cultural attitudes and practices – think how TikTok trends directly correlate with cosmetic surgery data, to name one sobering example.

What does this digital and cultural marginalisation look like in practice? When we assess the economic value of women, their primacy as consumers in an online empire built upon the profiteering of consumption, we know that being performatively female is an inherently lucrative cog in a money-making machine. This creates a cycle by which high profile women with large followers are banking on an effeminised identity which is then mined and sold back to us as a product. The highlighter which creates the 'cold girl' look or the 'boyfriend blush', made possible due to the very idea of female youth and beauty, exhibited via youth and beauty, and sold to us as such via conglomerates, all in time for the next recurrent trend, and the next ring of the perpetually moving till. Women are coerced into the drudgery of the consumer cycle via online spaces which make lots of people, lots of money.

And despite women's key role in online spaces – despite the fact that Instagram became the giant it is today arguably because of the make-up tutorial itself – women are consigned to the role of 'influencer' while men online occupy the title of 'creator'. Whole online empires are created off the back of anti-female sentiment and the online world is fuelled by unregulated hate towards women. The very disparities in how male – and female-domains are perceived is only further exemplified through the digisphere, despite how much of it rests upon and is built up by women. By the very values it propagates, the online world discredits women. It breeds the kind of ideology that leads to widespread anti-female sentiment that ruptures into the offline world. And this is not even to mention the dark underbelly of this internet, an Only Fans culture which has ruined the lives of, and continues to degrade, tens of thousands of women.

When we look at Muslim online spaces, similar dynamics exist. Whole armies of alt-right communities, and those vulnerable to right-wing thinking, are mobilised by cheap, easy and clearly fabricated 'calls for shariah/they're cancelling Christmas'-bait that awaken such existential angst. Additionally, the blue-and-white washing by companies with clear investments in genocide, and which faced successful boycott campaigns amongst Muslims, were the first to co-opt Muslim influencers to launder their image and repair the sizeable dent in their margins. Again, demonstrating how ripe the Muslim consumer is for exploitation, without any real accompanying regard for their rights or welfare. Corporations and individuals are happy to profit from Muslims, but far less likely to interrogate cultural biases, nor contribute materially or through meaningful dialogue towards their parity. These contradictions give us an insight into how the online world has, for many communities, created both regressive, as well as progressive, advancements.

The material impact of all of this hate – against women, Muslims, and in the ultimate intersection in the Venn Diagram of social illegitimacy, the Muslim woman herself – should not be underestimated. The memes, comment sections, morning talk show topics, legacy media headlines, click-bait digital headlines, hashtags, Substack articles – the storm cloud of hate-content under which many of us live, undoubtedly contributes to an increasingly hostile climate which makes life harder for the everyday Muslim, and visibly Muslim woman, in public life.

Ironically, much of Muslim social media's cultural needle is itself stuck on gender divisions. And as with everything that originates from the online world, it impacts real world impressions. This is particularly the case for Muslim mothers, whose very identity within the community is used as both a punishment and cure for Muslim women en masse. The Muslim mother is held up by Muslim communities online as the ultimate role, destiny, fulfilment for Muslim women, despite the lack of real-world support she receives from the community at large. And as we've already covered, this cultural hagiography which elevates the 'Mother' to superhuman standards does not benefit Muslim mums or women as a whole. If the sanctification of motherhood in broader culture exists, then in Muslim culture we see an attempt to elevate that pedestal.

For Muslim women, the social expectations projected on to us will have their own cultural cadences and those will have intra-community nuances; our racial, cultural, ethnic and even linguistic diversity means we are subject to different social environments and therefore slightly different conceptions and misconceptions regarding motherhood in Islam, depending on that cultural background. As a massively heterogenous community there are few commonalities in Muslim diaspora cultures and we are not, as a community, taking on the cultural baton from a monolithic Boomer generation like many others. However, due to a growing digital literacy, and an increase in how much of our thoughts and lives are influenced and consumed by the online world, there is a single, converging expectation of Muslim women created by a homogenised internet culture made up of a new digital generation of Muslim men. Muslim women are subsequently being subjected to a universal kind of pressure, originally borne from these digital channels. Very often, this means you are likely to come across a kind of expectation of you based specifically on your identity as a Muslim mum in particular, a kind of strange possessive net that absolute strangers will attempt to cast over you, using Islam to justify their intrusions.

As such, despite our world of ever changing ideals, economic uncertainty and technological advancement – one thing remains stubbornly consistent. Online Muslim discourse. While the world around us charges ahead, you are guaranteed to find IslamLove786 versus an obscure-pop-culture-reference Twitter/ X handle stuck in a fierce debate as to whether or not Muslim women should 'stay at home'. This fixation with gender roles, which very often is borne from a misogyny entirely incompatible with Islam, is otherwise quite telling. As Muslims with essentialist gender values, at a time when gender is such a hotly-contest subject, it is no wonder that such debate is so fiercely ignited. For a community which is so beautifully diverse, there are few issues we huddle around the collective fire of so greatly, than gender – it is often a universal consideration for young Muslims, our own lingua franca so to speak. This more so because of the homogenisation of young Muslim men around alt-right, 'Alpha-male' social media figures who make tenuous claim to Islamic values. Also, as a community which by-and-large is homosocial, these debates expose a kind of immaturity concerning the very topic of gender relations – which it is worth saying, is *not* natural to Islam – but which can lead to incendiary, puerile views which invite attention and chatter.

Our perennial obsession with gender relations in Islam exposes both the retrogressive and innovative currents of internet culture – in how Muslims are being sold a lie of gender traditionalism in Islam, on the basis of a modern format of misogyny.

And it all started with the Incel.

Not MINC-ing words

It's hard to describe Incel, and Red Pill culture, to the uninitiated. Though much of its own demographic are now too young to acknowledge, Red Pill as a term and movement is a cultural reference to a key moment in modern cinema. The Fin De Sciele period is that historic time, at the end of a century, when social angst is brought to the fore. During the turn of the century, in late Victorian literature, we saw a similar ideological tussle play itself out in the novels of the day. As we approach a new epoch in human history, humanity self-flagellates about all that came before and all that might, or might not, lie ahead. The Matrix, a film made in 1999, and in which the term 'Red Pill's allegorical roots lie, similarly speaks to that culture of Millenium panic and uncertainty. That one of the most panic-stricken movements in cultural history borrows from this film is very fitting.

Much like its political opposite of 'woke', the term Red Pill denotes a kind of social and political awakening. It references the choice the main character in The Matrix was given, in the projected alternative reality in which he inhabited – a choice between swallowing a red pill that will allow him to learn the hard truth about the world in which he lives, and a blue pill that will allow him to stay oblivious and return to his normal life of simulation and delusion. Similarly, Red Pillers and Incels believe that capitalist patriarchy, and male privilege, is a social mirage that they've just awoken from, which masks a deeply misandrist society.

Conversely, these male-supremacist movements have constructed, and are now fully immersed in, an alternative reality in which they believe female privilege overwhelmingly shackles men to positions of disadvantage, socially, economically and romantically. Red Pillers are intellectually superior to both women and 'blue pill normies' who are still in denial of this apparent truth of a female-world-order. According to the proponents of this inverted truth, the interests of women dictate social and political systems, leaving men longhoused, marginalised and discriminated against. This is despite the very material evidence we have which states the opposite. Incel communities, which started life as esoteric movements on rarefied websites such as Reddit and 4chan, have diffused into a kind of normalised misogyny, beyond the manosphere, and into mainstream iterations of the web – primarily through the vehicle of podcast bros and YouTubers. These cyberculture enclaves act as ideological havens for aggrieved men who believe they are downtrodden by the force of female entitlement. Indeed, the very term 'incel' is a portmanteau built from the terms 'Involuntary Celibate' referring to the defining feature of these male communities. They display romantic frustrations because they consider themselves unable to attract women – a fact which communicates both their sense of entitlement and victimhood to the world. Inceldom is effectively this plaintive cry for an apparently lost world-order which privileges men.

Worryingly, this movement has made violent protrusions into the real world in the shape of increasingly misogynistic attitudes, abuse against women and, at the extreme end of the scale, an ultimate "Black Pill" culture of mass shootings and other violent hate crimes.

In reality, Inceldom and Red Pill thought is the result of the social anxiety that exists around the role of male identity in these volatile economic times. As the nuclear 'Fordian' family, the white picket-fence dream, becomes obsolete, and the traditional gender and economic roles that define it face threats from social, political, cultural and global shifts to its foundations, the gender orthodoxy which hallmark capitalist societies is left disfigured.

What does this have to do with the Muslim man?

While political powers depend upon a vilified Muslim identity in order to justify the industrial-complexes on which they depend, the Muslim identity will always be ripe for exploitation and manipulation. Is it any wonder, then, that Inceldom has found such healthy expression in the online Muslim world. This tortured social alchemy creating a proud army of Mincels; 'Muslim involuntarily celibate men'.

There are a number of factors which result in young Muslim men being so taken by this inherently racist and sexist ideology which, not insignificantly, was borne from white, Christian, male culture – hitherto top of the global food chain. During these increasingly uncertain social and economic times, Muslim families – and questions pertaining to gender roles in the Muslim home – face similar contestations. This environment of uncertainty is similarly generating existential discomfort amongst Muslim men for whom bedrocks of masculinity such as marriage and economic primacy are no longer at arm's reach, creating an identity crisis which sees Muslim men aggressively assume exaggerated and superficial qualities of masculinity as defence. A lack of religious literacy amongst men, and women, who have an elementary grasp of Islam, is similarly a massive contributory factor to the consolidation of such movements. As are erroneous mainstream ideas of manliness which dictate to us that 'piety' doesn't sit comfortably with modern conceptions of masculinity – and which associate liberal approaches to relationships and promiscuity; an ambivalence and detachment, as hallmarks of manliness. This is why Mincel role models will compulsively assume these secular notions of masculinity as window dressing to qualify or balance their expressed faith that the world at large has wrongly effeminised.

For men who have been fed lies and fallacies about their religion, Incel is an attractive prospect. Which brings us on to the second, more pertinent, push factor of this alarming trend. Internalised Islamophobia is another significant driver of this currency of misogyny amongst young Muslim men; as the Muslim identity is increasingly problematised, Muslims by default are placed on the back foot, qualifying Islam through a secular, non-Muslim lens; attaching it to symbols of perceived greatness to make up for its perceived deficiencies. With the racialised make-up of Muslims in the West, there are also many racial nuances that further complicate this unfortunate tendency – whitewashing for legitimacy is synonymous with secularisation in the Muslim world.

The validation that young Muslim men seek is satiated when WASP (White Anglo-Saxon Protestant) culture, and its most prominent media figures, wrongly attribute, and glorify, a whole range of racist, orientalist and Islamophobic tropes to Islam and Muslims. They wrongly redeem these ideas of themselves, as Muslim men – on false bases – for example being abjectly misogynistic and emotionally absent from their wives and children. In effect, Muslim men have begun to accept false and crude stereotypes regarding Islamic masculinity that are being celebrated by burgeoning online communities, as they are reclaimed as part of Western tradition and heralded as the way forward. Even the glorification of such traits and qualities is a kind of subordination for the Muslim man, as it is the non-Muslim endorsement of them which grants them this appeal and shiny veneer. For this generation of young Muslim men who were forced into the role of cultural pariahs – this represents a shift in a value system that has always had them in a chokehold, and which now presents an opportunity for cultural redemption. Coupled with lazy political thinking which creates a false alliance between right-wing and Muslim interests in popular Muslim thought, and the cultural ground becomes fertile for the rapid growth of this ideology.

The attention economy on which digital content thrives means that naturally, Muslim male influencers are now taking on and glibly promoting the ideological cadences of this internet movement that glamourises sexual and domestic violence. The convolution between misogyny and Islam is so cemented in modern Muslim thought, that anti-female views become the basis by which social media influencers lay their claim to Islam – it has become a mark of Islamic authenticity in the dawah world to speak disparagingly of the idea of female rights, without any curiosity as to what that means for the women in these men's lives, or the Muslim women that are impacted by their words. In fact many non-Muslim social media personalities who eventually convert to Islam are initiated through misogyny – their endorsing of "traditional gender" roles becomes what they are identified as being 'Muslim adjacent' for. It is very troubling that anti-female sentiment has such a great mindshare amongst prominent, social media Muslims today, as are the implications of this for a generation of impressionable audiences. These high-profile digital figures, who directly profiteer off culture wars, are drawn towards the reactive Muslim audience and all the lucrative benefits they may bring.

This wider migration creates an impression that Muslim men, who are increasingly shaping our online appetites, have a greater sense of loyalty to men – Muslim and non – than Muslim women themselves. Indeed, much of the extreme behaviour that Incel movements foment are caused by 'identity fusion' – a sense of oneness felt by individuals within a group or movement that results in personally costly, extreme pro-group behaviours. Mincel offers Muslim men a kind of visceral connection to this fraternity, which comes at the expense of their relationship with their families and their Muslim sisters in Islam.

As a community we appear to be willingly donning the monstrous mask of Islamophobic caricatures, now placated by social media influencers. These influencers, who are clocking up tens of thousands of hits and are increasingly legitimised, appear to revel in the subversive nature of their anti-female views, apparently unaware that the identity they occupy is just as much a making of secular ideology as the feminism they claim to be fighting a righteous battle against.

Muslim men who have been conscripted by this false doctrine are equally pacified by the reassuringly simple narrative that they propagate, and which provides a welcome distraction from the complexities of real life. When you are vilified in the media, when economic milestones are more challenging, falling back on an aggrandised male identity which grants you social capital is a tempting prospect.

Real life examples of how this is harming Muslim women, mothers and their children are endless. Emotionally and physically abusive relationships are all but celebrated online – and disturbing narratives coming directly from Muslim men – who are expressly comparing women to *shaitan*

– are promoting the mistreatment of women, erroneously in the name of Islamic ideology. The impression that the more the Muslim man revels in the subjugation, emotional detachment and alienation of his wife, the healthier the relationship according to Islamic norms, has become embedded in some prominent Muslim male online cultures, and is trickling into the psyche of many young, impressionable Muslim men who see this content as religiously affirming. One haunting example of what's celebrated as Muslim male behaviour – apparently within the confines of Islam – includes a Muslim man boasting about his partner delivering their child alone, and serving him tea directly after – revelling in the subjugation of a physically and emotionally vulnerable woman. Others include not providing financial support to their wives, or manipulating their finances to disadvantage them, of refusing to fulfil the Sunnah of helping in the home as though that is an additional armour of masculinity. Ironically, these attitudes are antithetical to the Prophetic tradition that Islam is built upon, which includes an honourable focus on empathy, compassion and charity – not to mention a whole moral code upon which marital relations and rights are honoured.

The construct of the punitive, harsh and corrective Muslim male in popular Muslim thought is simultaneously and contradictorily portrayed as both the result of divine law and natural order, and as a punishing measure for the straying of Muslim women. Where 'straying' is often Muslim women seeking basic rights that Islam itself has afforded her.

In reality, one could ask oneself whether it is Muslim women that should be lamenting the loss of Islamic masculinity, through social tantrums, or otherwise. This emptying of Islamic masculinity is exemplified in how the Muslim manosphere reduces complex, socially driven principles of Shariah to objects of male desire – be it polygamy, or the *fiqh* [26] around marriage and divorce. The terms of debate regarding polygamy, for example, are crudely shaped entirely by male desire, and the social responsibility, which a majority of scholars classify as the purpose of multiple marriages, remains an invisible and neglected consideration. In fact, the entire premise of this noble tradition has been embroiled in scabrous locker-room talk, which is used by prominent online Muslim men under the ostensible aim of asserting religious normativism, but which works as a cover to grant

---

[26] Islamic jurisprudence

them clout and street cred. A street cred which it appears they feel is more native to Islam than honouring the Muslim woman – these men appear to have internalised, and are now inhabiting, a barometer of masculinity which is antithetical to Islam.

Many male, Muslim social media personalities appear to approach the table with the kind of arrogance and moral grandstanding that is both antithetical to the demeanour of our beloved Prophet ﷺ and which naturally reviles Muslim women who they claim to be also speaking in the interests of. They are further supported by a wider group of Muslim men who appear to be oblivious to the hurt caused on both an individual, micro level, and on a macro level, and who are, at best, heavy-handed in their approach to promoting Islamic edicts, or at worse, actively exploiting it to justify spiritual and physical abuse. This digital manifestation, casts a real life shadow in many of the lives of Muslim mums, and needs to be unequivocally driven out of our real and online spaces.

Our own internal algorithm

Mincel figures and those Muslim social media personalities adjacent to them are building the castles of their fiefdom atop of this Islamophobic digital landscape. As a group, they are trading in a dangerous world of symbolism which builds upon and therefore consolidates the idea of Islam as an illicit belief and subaltern practice. In an online world fuelled by user-generated content, and shaped entirely by popular consumption and instinctive drive, social media acts as a black mirror to our deepest whims, desires, quirks and aspirations. Internet traffic shaped by our habits reveal curiosities and traits unknown even to us. Since its inception, the internet has been our closest confidant, we reveal more to the Google search engine, and are known more intimately by our TikTok for you pages, than even our closest friends. Our relationship with the internet is now more dysfunctional than ever – as it is speaking to, and directly feeding off, our most latent and base self, one that works on millisecond impulses, and like a petulant and overindulged child, demands stimuli. We are effectively creating a living breathing hive of content from the unearthed pits of our minds. This then forms the basis of the content we live our lives by, forming our cultural consciousness. This back and forth relationship between our online appetite and consumption creates an unhealthy, and increasingly degenerative, feedback loop. Content created by Muslims with large audiences is therefore both a reflection of our collective psychology as Muslims, and can tap into that same hinterland of space when it shapes and sets new norms.

Muslim influencers – knowingly or not – are fuelled by this subconscious resource – an algorithm which is shaped by, and shapes, our own subconscious biases. This trench of collective thought is the site for all those repressed ideas we collate regarding Islam, from the discards of popular media, news and culture, and often in place of true knowledge regarding our faith. As such, there is a burgeoning, and commonly exploitative trend, whereby Muslim influencers appear to use outward expressions of faith – and symbols of 'Muslimness' – for the attention and clout they have accrued from centuries of 'illicitness', made more translatable in the online world. This in turn creates a lucrative form of engagement.

It produces a kind of pantomime of Muslimness in which influencers appear to revel in the supposedly subversive nature of the Muslim identity, using the illicit connotations of Islam in overt and covert ways. They extrapolate orthodox beliefs and practices, for example, and use the crude stage of social media platforms to showcase them in ways that rid them of context, nuance and theology. This is done entirely to attention farm; to engage

Islamophobic vitriol in rage-bait purely for the clicks, and to capture Muslim audiences who have falsely internalised the dichotomy we spoke of in the previous chapter, and who want to 'reclaim' religion on that false basis. Producing and engaging in this kind of content provides them with a false badge of heroism and valour, giving them the unearned title of defenders of faith. Often, these creators are basically oiling the wheels of Islamophobia and cementing illicit impressions of Islam, and content of this nature will end up being shared and replicated on both corners of the "splinternet" – in right-wing, flag-bearing profiles, and amongst Muslims. A bear-baiting which has created a strange shared cultural relish between these two opposing worlds, and which grants these content makers twice the bang for their internet buck. This dog whistle to secular audiences, which frames the very notion of Islam as ludicrous and absurd, is received as a nod to less socially and political astute Muslim viewers who seek the kind of paltry validation that comes from mainstream referencing.

This digital language is a kind of hybrid messaging that simultaneously speaks to two opposing audiences. A strange, shadowy double-speak which achieves both aims that appear to preoccupy the Muslim manosphere – the first, of appearing masculine according to secular barometers of masculinity, and the second, to be deemed adequately Islamic as "Islamic" is culturally coded through superficial symbols. It represents the strange convergence of Red Pill misogyny and Islam that we see through digital, male expressions of Muslim male identity, and exposes the very contradictions which underpin the meeting of these two constructs. It exposes the very issue concerning algorithmic influence on our private impressions and public performance of faith. And of course it exemplifies the strange and superficial relationship we develop with social media personalities, with whom we have the kind of digital proximity which harbours parasocial sentiment, and which leaves us open to obvious manipulation. For Muslim mums this includes tropes and figures we will go on to discuss.

One example of this phenomenon is content creators using their polygamous relationships, and symbols like the niqab, and garnering audiences based on the intrigue and sense of illegitimacy surrounding these practices. Their very sense of pride in these credibly Islamic traditions is rooted in the notion that these ideas are almost socially forbidden and interdicted, and our reception of them as Muslim audiences becomes more and more divorced from the scripture in which they're rooted. We begin to measure their authentic claim to Islam via how malformed they are to secular sensibilities – and appear to feel validated by the bone of social media approval we are thrown. Critically, it creates a dual coding of Islam as subversive, and acceptable on account of its subversion alone. And it is precisely what Mincel's protagonists bank on when creating this kind of content. Resultantly, expressions of Muslimness, like the niqab, come to accumulate these added cultural dimensions – droll and outlandish. These symbols are therefore rewritten in our cultural cannon according to these reductive scripts, and take on their belittling and shameful cadences. The material impact of which on the most visibly Muslim demographic – niqabi women – is a shameful indictment of an industry of supposedly pro-Islamic content.

There is something inherently incompatible between this Mincel content and Islam. Both the metric by which Mincel is celebrated – secular concepts of male acquisition – and the mode by which its celebrated – fickle and anachronistic social media approval – are hostile grounds for true faith or practice. It exemplifies how redundant social media is as a medium to discuss nuanced *fiqh* positions in Islam that require further thought, and not impulsive reactions.

When we turn our already very misunderstood faith practices into TikTok content, we do them a disservice – we quash and reduce the rich, theological and historical traditions on which they are based and reduce them to shallow fodder for entertainment alone. The popular impressions of our faith practices also suffer from a wider phenomenon in the online world, what cultural critics term the 'generation loss' – when the same content is generated repeatedly, a form of degradation occurs that corrupts the information, and compromises on its quality. This process of generation loss is inbuilt to technologies of the digital age and leads to what theorists describe as a 'cultural doom loop'.[xlviii] The cultural signals of Muslimness that make up popular internet content, that achieve virality and are then repeated by a number of influencers, cement faulty impressions that are only further falsified through repeated interpretations by content creators keen to get their own slice of the internet infamy pie. The sum result is a marked attrition of our faith impressions.

This downward spiral my also explain the deplorable social media debates in and around the Mincel space that have brought us paradoxes such as 'temporary' and 'one minute nikkah's, and

'McDonalds as *Mahr*'[27] reference points which further denigrates Muslim women – whose apparent honour justifies the entire Mincel endeavour – and of course Islamic practice. They also expose a new generation of young, impressionable Muslim men to the supposed religious legitimacy of temporary marriages with fast-food pay outs. This perpetual cycle of content also neglects to even acknowledge women as possessing any religious intellectual appetite, and actively attempts to sacrifice our *imaan* in the sycophantic quest for secular Incel approval. When Muslim men and women weigh up their options, these flippant anecdotes shape their understanding of Islam – both in terms of *fiqh*, and our perceptions of what is deemed proper and improper conduct and engagement.

Crucially, if we become accustomed to dealing in symbols of illicitness, when it comes to understanding and practising our faith, we are effectively excommunicating it from its true origin of scripture and the intent to please Allāh. What the manosphere is ignorant of is its complicity with a wider Islamophobic culture which works to deform and delegitimise our faith. This creates a kind of schizophrenic morality that is incon-

---

27 Dower

gruous with true Islam and therefore our very fitrah. As an audience we are looking up to them purely on the basis that they are 'counter-culture' alone, and not because they are done for the sake of Allāh. As such, the more they signal deformity to non-Muslim audiences, the more we feel validated and assuaged. We are effectively shaping our understanding of Islam around the verboten black space of the internet, creating our own warped internal algorithm. As Muslims, we are hamstrung by our total lack of understanding of Islam outside of these dark, digital manifestations. True Islamic practice becomes a heterodox to the sense of it perpetuated online; we begin to see our faith as at odds with a scripture that speaks to us with more compassion and nuance than the internet has the capacity to bear in its current iteration. Muslim mums, and our children, are being fed and are developing increasingly warped notions of our faith, carried by a self-worsening herd mentality.

Girl power?

The Muslim community has been slow to respond to Mincel culture, despite its worrying size and pace of growth, and its obvious harms on the Muslim home. And many community figures that have addressed it have sadly attributed it to a rise in feminism amongst Muslim women. While the underlying reasons for the sprouting of Inceldom in Muslim digital spaces are complex, including a misogyny inherent in some Muslim cultures themselves, the insistence within the Muslim community of lazily ascribing the popularity of these movements to 'feminism' – in short, women – does nothing to address or remedy this distressing trend. In fact, it mirrors the wider pattern amongst the Inceldom beyond the Muslim world, where there is an insistence on portraying Red Pill communities as fighting a righteous cultural war against feminism. We are effectively affirming their own deluded narrative. A narrative which paradoxically posits the woman as inferior, but capable of possessing the ultimate power – to manipulate the entire world's men to her end.

In the eyes of incels, the feminist is the ultimate evil and the main cause of their social demise. Equally, amongst Red Pill apologists, the idea of the 'feminist'/ liberal Muslim woman is presented as the sole driver for men involuntarily being pushed into hateful stances. It is worrying that despite the recognition that Red Pill thought is antithetical to Islam, we are seeing a constant excusing of poor Muslim, male behaviour.

This false equivalence between feminism and Inceldom is itself another contradictory dimension to Inceldom – the former is an intellectual, political and social movement spanning centuries, borne from an extended history of abuse and inequality, and the latter an undesirable and unintelligible internet off-shoot based on self-victimisation. This posturing does little to address the gravity of the situation at hand.

The gender debates that occupy Muslim men and women are tellingly based on suppositions about our own religion, which are entirely reactive and false. Just like the answers to social unease amongst Muslim men cannot be found in secular or non-Muslim solutions, the expression of this social angst should unequivocally not mirror that of non-Muslim, or unIslamic cultures like Red Pill. In the same way that conventional gender roles in Muslim and non-Muslim, Western culture are in no way aligned, Muslim men cannot hark back to a history of gender norms that do not belong to Islamic culture. They should not interpret Red Pill as a rallying cry of solidarity from men across the globe; their aims and motivations are not the same. Islamic masculinity comes from a place of security and *taqwā*, not insecurity and panic.

Equally, the reductive and patently false flag of 'Islam is a feminist religion' itself does Islam a disservice – Islam, a divine moral code set by our Creator, will always be transcendentally and substantively more than any humanly defined phenomenon. Islam established women's God-given rights as equal believers, and exists as a universal truth that outspans any earthly social movement and its claims to parity or equity. The need for Muslim women to lay claim to feminism as a means of equal treatment speaks of the conceptual dwarfing of Islam in Western intellect, and the mistreatment of Muslim women in Muslim societies. Indeed it also speaks to how the converse is true, and how 'feminism' becomes inflated to include any perceived act of dissent from women, and how this can be as small as expressing an opinion or wanting a voice. In all, it speaks of an utter confusion, and sometimes deliberate perversion, of what it means to be a Muslim woman.

If the Muslim feminist is continually touted as the ultimate evil, and feminism itself attributed to female ungodliness, then as a community we need to address why Incel culture is repeatedly spoken about as an inevitable response to feminism, and not men being just as prone to unIslamic ideologies. We need to unpack why an entirely male phenomenon is being attributed to women. And why Muslim women clutching onto secular models of equality is not seen in the same victimised way – despite the shameful mountain of statistical evidence which demonstrates that a worrying number of women are on the receiving end of physical, emotional and spiritual abuse in our communities.

Taken to its logical conclusion, this line of argument which assigns no blame to men implies that men are morally infallible, and women inherently corrupt. This reasoning reinforces the most ugly tenets of Red Pill thinking and creates an ideal environment for the continued abuse of women to thrive. It is especially damaging given women are overwhelmingly the victim of Red Pill and Incel culture, not men; it is in essence ideological victim blaming. It shifts the onus onto women and encourages further self-victimisation amongst men who are developing increasingly warped perceptions of reality. It exposes the revolving door that our communities have created between Incel culture and Muslim communities.

The undercurrents of this thinking, the idea of the original female sin and the morally reprehensible woman, are as old as time and as alien to Islam as the Red Pill ideology they prop up and support. They demonstrate the disfigured, ahistorical Islam that is adopted by men in these movements, and are worsening a situation whose only cure is to return to the Quran and Sunnah, and for men to adopt the sense of responsibility, honour, accountability and kindness that characterised our Prophet ﷺ.

While this apologism collectively allows Muslim men, and the hateful male spaces that exist within them, to evade responsibility – and does nothing to advance the lost masculinity they claim to mourn – individually it does young Muslim men a great disservice. It grants them an impunity that does them a disfavour as believers particularly, and denies them the opportunity for self-reflection and growth. When young men see prominent figures in the community defer accountability for the wrongs of Mincel onto Muslim women, they are effectively being told not to assume any duty or obligation as Muslim men – it is entirely emasculating. In keeping with a more general trend in Muslim cultures of disburdening men from responsibility, it stunts their moral development and prevents them from reaching their potential. If our moral well being depends upon an unadulterated relationship with reality and our own selves – then perhaps we ought to be questioning what cultural and religious leaders achieve by cushioning men from these social, economic and personal blows.

Unfortunately it is in keeping with the ideological migration we see of furthering away from the Sunnah. While the grounds of the debate continues to shift to more extreme positions, we risk alienating more and more women, while they face further individual and collective scrutiny in demanding their basic rights as believers. As a community, and particularly for Muslim men, we need to understand that misogyny, the ideological bedfellow of Islamophobia, is a characteristic of the forefathers of anti-Muslim sentiment, the Quraish, and should be eschewed by the inheritors of our faith. It is without doubt an inherent trait of the Jahil.

Old misogyny in Muslim Cultures

I often wonder what would happen if women assumed as a baseline the confidence of a man who's never cooked a day in his life, yet offers unsolicited feedback on others women's cooking. While such self-certitude is arguably quite admirable, the heritage-misogyny that leads to these interesting quirks in our cultural experiences do need to be challenged. Because it does become incumbent upon us as Muslims to assert the truth of our faith outside of these modern constructs sold to us as authentic Islam. It bears mentioning here, therefore, the existing template of anti-female sentiment that exists in Muslim cultures, and which, due to our linear understanding of history, and black and white notion of geography and culture, is fiercely guarded in the name of 'traditionalism', and wrongly seen as tantamount to Islam. We have seen the issues caused by the racialisation of Islam, and are often vocal opponents of it, yet we ourselves often fall into lazy habits of equating customs indigenous to Eastern culture as unquestioningly Islamic. This blanket acceptance of anything "culturally Muslim" as "Islamic" further obscures our impressions of Islam, which is a conscious and purposeful endeavour, not an acceptance of any one tradition or culture for its sake alone. And we know a human pattern of behaviour which, like a knot weed, is stubbornly consistent and culturally resolute, and which our own Prophet ﷺ warned us against – is the continuing denigration of women.

Sentiments which fall under this tradition that we see in South Asian and in some Arab cultures, which are thankfully not exhaustive of the Muslim world, is a menacing paradox in which men are considered so sacrosanct they can't perform the qualifying tasks to assume this 'sacred' status. In these cultures, men are sometimes deemed so precious that they're freed of all the typically 'male' responsibility. This is naturally transferred to women, who are burdened with the additional responsibility – the emotional and physical toll – but none of the status or recognition. Conversely they're punished for it. Not only is this contrary to Islam but it creates this strange social mirage that we all blindly inhabit, in which men are increasingly 'effeminised' under the emperors robes of an empty masculinity – giving them the throne but none of the noble features deserving of it – and women are 'masculinised' to accommodate and make up for that social shortfall.

Effectively men are rewarded by a femininity that is both denied to women, and which women are beaten down for not having the luxury to take advantage of. And that same 'male' domain and social value that women are effectively assuming is devalued by its association with women. What this does on a macro level we are seeing via Red Pill and all its variants, what it does in the micro is leave women increasingly vulnerable but having to assume a strength they are then berated for.

This is reflective of the secular trends in Inceldom which found such rapid breeding ground in Muslim communities. When popular, mainstream, and highly followed Incels speak about the erosion of family values – they frame the same ills they identify as the downfall of traditionalism as the punishment for that crime. For example, pornography is bad and leading to moral corruption – therefore we should subjugate women through this industry further. This is particularly the case from some high-profile Incel personalities who have active interests in the adult entertainment industries. This enables them to deflect any responsibility for their shortcomings onto the female victims of this industry, it means they don't have the arduous moral straightjacket of sticking to their principles, and are basically able to practise the opposite of what they preach, and remain unaccountable.

And this concept dovetails well into cultural approaches to gender in Muslim households. It therefore appeals to some men who grew up in Muslim families, as they can equally externalise guilt and responsibility. They can assume the veneer of respectability without having to adhere to any principles. It is benevolent patriarchy without the benevolence or the patriarch. Holding extremist views on gender is, according to this ideology, the ultimate badge of honour and elevates them to the status of defenders of traditional values and respectability without any of the necessary work or effort, particularly not on themselves. These movements and the personalities that lead and profiteer from them, wittingly or not, have tapped into a special kind of religious guilt and inferiority complex that lies latent in some Muslim cultures, eviscerated of Islam. And they are now reaping the benefits of awakening this cultural poltergeist through clicks and likes and all the eventual profit that brings. And Muslim audiences are paying most greatly for this through their very faith.

The gender imbalance in some Muslim communities is manifest in the everyday, reinforced by both men and women, through the standards we expect of girls, versus those of Muslim boys – the well-recorded over-achievement of Muslim women in families where Muslim men are pandered into ineffectiveness. Take, for example, how 'growth' becomes a gendered concept – women are expected to endure, inure, adapt so that men can remain in their apparent sacrosanct natural state. Or regress further into it. It is hard to tell if we – as a community of both men and women – are collectively infantilising men because society loves them and thinks they deserve a life of domestic ease, or because we are creating industries of work for women because we are scared of their potential outside of domesticity. What is becoming more apparent is that we, as a community in our entirety, are celebrating an empty masculinity rather than encouraging a Prophetic one, at the expense of women. Very often we are still applauding the concept of Man, despite the Prophetic qualities no longer being present or even encouraged.

In particular, what unites these old institutions of misogyny with their newer, digital counterparts, is the unique punishment they reserve for divorced women and single mothers in particular, exposing an insecurity concerning the very foundational role a man should assume in Islam. Premised on what we can only assume is the idea that men qualify women – a presumption necessary of course because there is no basis for this disdain in Islam itself – many contemporary popular dawah figures uphold a punitive spectrum which shamefully places divorced women and single mothers on the undeserving and illegitimate end of this already very ignoble imaginary scale.

This thinking upholds a kind of puritanical view of divorce as shameful, and places that shame and apparent dishonour entirely at the door of the woman. It works on the assumption that men are inherently faultless, and worthy of second chances

– indeed perennial 'first chances' as they are deemed unblemished by divorce. This is of course paradoxical, given the digital popular dawah world's obsession with 'temporary marriages' – an illegitimate concept in mainstream Islam – a driver for the divorce they insist on punishing women for.

Often marriage is used as a kind of rotten carrot to contrast the stick of an unIslamic lifestyle. As though the male-issued reward for 'pious' women is a commitment in marriage. This is despite Mincel in particular just stopping short of publishing actual guides on how to subjugate their wives and deny them any of the spousal support mandatory in Islam. This anti-female, unIslamic sentiment tells on itself time and time again; there is no qualifying feature a woman can assume, Islamic or otherwise, that grants these figurative women they frame as 'marriage worthy', the honour they position themselves to bequeath. In fact, it is based entirely on a kind of male-centric view which is posited on the very idea that specifically a man's feelings and thoughts are what bequeath women status in religion. As though their very approval is what authorises women's success in religious terms.

This misogyny which is shared by traditional and newer strains of thinking is almost always presupposed on the idea of the woman as an insentient object. Situated entirely in secular and pre-Islamic concepts of relationships, which position women as mere accessories for men's social and physical gratification, this damaging strain of thinking privileges male bodily pleasures and exonerates men of any sense of duty to the women in their lives, and indeed of any blame – both of which are antithetical to Islam.

That these views and the exploitation of women they encourage are so popular in the digital age is a testament to the strength of their foundations in the non-digital world that precedes it. It also underscores one of the prevailing themes of this book – the false binaries upon which we lazily base our religious impressions. Many Muslim men, on and offline, will, as discussed, see themselves as defenders of a tradition they perceive as obverse to 'Western' culture. The digital manifestations of this sense of conventionalism that we see in the popular dawah industry, is actually a skilful weaving together of the unIslamic elements of both Eastern and Western culture while maintaining the PR of Muslimness, by exploiting the binary ideas we have concerning both worlds.

Though we can say, unequivocally, it is not all Muslim men, and though we can, rightly, speak against any blanket hate directed at Muslim men, what we must also recognise is how these cultures will colour all of us in different ways. We must also be cognisant of the cyclical nature of culture whereby we are so unnerved by uprooting the cultural norms that sit outside Islam, that we are so devoted to. This sense of nervous gate-keeping of ideals when we see new cultural values and practices in a succeeding generation exists because it reminds us so acutely that the norms we cherish, and invest so much of ourselves in, are themselves constructed, unnatural – and at one point in the hamster wheel of history, themselves new and subversive. They also expose this strange place many Muslims inhabit in the nexus of time and place – for many diaspora Muslims, for example, the idea of Islam is a traditionalism that is crystalised in the customs of their parents' home during the time those parents still inhabited it. We are wed to certain ideas that are inextricably linked to their time and place in history, and which our nostalgia and tribalism wants us to hold on to. As Muslims, with fidelity to the truth, we need to interrogate these illegitimate strains of thinking that we often wrongly deem as authentic, through the lens of Islam.

The very language around Islam as 'backwards' that we vocally oppose but internally affirm in many ways is itself telling of our perception of our faith as something stubbornly rooted in time. Islam is a timeless ideology – as Muslims we do not affirm or negate anything on the basis of its time, we do so on its truth. There are practices that are deemed 'regressive' that we may be inclined to denounce on that basis alone, and there are others we see as 'progressive' that those who think in a counter way will reject on this basis alone too. The centre point in both these directional references is of course a secular humanism, based on Enlightenment ideals. The barometer through which we measure truth should be uncompromisingly the Quran and Sunnah.

It is an interesting time for gender dynamics in as far as how ideals for men have rightly evolved, while those for women remain static. There's now a lot more understanding and sympathy for the stereotypical role of the breadwinner and also the idea of appearing stoic and emotionally impermeable, but this isn't mirrored in the treatment or expectation of women whose domestic labour is considered a limitless resource and who are still expected to carry a lot of emotional burden. Indeed, much of what constitutes modern day 'nagging' is basically women bargaining for space in a world that seeks to limit and define it. The original binaries of public/private and professional/domestic that women and men are supposed to assume, in a world where those distinctions are blurred, are not necessarily always healthy, nor are they unquestioningly aligned with Islam, however this current iteration, and the hypocrisy that underlies it, is in need of address.

Out of the Matrix...

The material harms of Mincel on Muslim mums is obvious – and this is in light of a growing femcel movement which indicates an increasing number of young girls and women themselves have bought into the Incel gender ideology; a fact which underscores the conversation necessary regarding women's role as mothers in shaping the Mincel... It has also led to a dismaying online trend where the Quran and Sunnah are quoted as a kind of one-up-man-ship between men and women, often times as though the point isn't to seek the truth – to find the right moral code by which to live our lives – rather it is to affirm an existing bias that we are blinkered by. So how do we extract ourselves from this gender deadlock which is dominating Muslim discussion and leading to men increasingly exonerating themselves from defining responsibilities, creating disharmony between Muslim men and women, and leading to discontent and broken marriages?

What we need to see is Muslim men unequivocally denouncing the Mincel movement which is part of an unrelenting course of punishing Muslim women that exists beyond our faith community with no geographical borders or limits. If Muslim women are the ideological punch bag of world leaders, domestic policy, and the wilderness of internet discourse and its material impact on our homes – then one might ask what hope we have of moving forward as a community, or more pertinently who might Muslim women be able to turn to if we are both the cause and victim to our apparently justified abuse?

The countless examples of the Prophet's ﷺ love, mercy, kindness, compassion and tenderness to the women in his life and in society at large should be the basis by which we begin the conversation on gender relations, given the wider climate of disparity. The well-known example of *Banu Qainuqa*, a Medinian tribe that dishonoured a Muslim woman and against whom the Prophet ﷺ lay siege for fifteen days as a result, goes some way in demonstrating the tradition of respecting and upholding the dignity of Muslim women in Islam.

There must be a concerted effort to finally decouple misogyny from Islam as it now exists in the minds of Muslim men and women, and to understand Islam not as an endorsement of or reaction to modern or pre-modern eras, but a timeless ideology which stands independently and which wholly recognises men and women as twin halves in faith. Muslim men need to be educated on our history, to fully recognise that misogyny is not a Muslim trait, and never has been. In the conventional social hierarchy, changes which birthed this screaming and distressed Red Pill movement, Muslim men sit far below the white men who promulgate this view. A defining feature of racist ideology is the pandering to men of colour who they deem as inferior, when it suits their misogynistic agenda. Muslim men, like women, are no more than a tool in the broader Incel manifesto.

Indeed, capitalism has a long history of dividing men and women in the name of labour efficiency. Men are socialised to seek companionship in homosocial environments that benefit capital, while the beauty industry sews a profitable distrust between women who will be swayed to seek that comradery in marital relations alone. Similarly, the gender and culture wars stoked between Muslim men and women only seek to undermine the foundations of the Muslim family.

The greatest love story we are sold is the one between man and product – consumerism is this romanticisation of consumption that pervades our everyday lives. If our gender identities as men and women are relational, then for an economic system which benefits from ruthless individualism, those relationships, and sense of value and collectiveness, are eroded by the natural grind of the capitalist machine.

The broader, global and generation-defining, political migration of men towards a kind of social conservatism, and women towards more progressive ideologies, is almost entirely mirrored in Muslim communities. It is indicative of our intellectual habits, now shaped by the dual-coded digital world, of subscribing to 'packages' of ideals, and the moral laziness and social cowardice of identarianism that accompanies it. South Korea, where these differences are most acute, appears to be a harbinger for the future, giving us a prescience into cultural issues to come. A country which is the subject of the world's intrigue due to its position as possessing the single lowest fertility rate in the world, and where men and women are increasingly on opposite ends of social, political, cultural and spatial divides. That we are passively and unquestioningly adopting sociopolitical identities as Muslims who mistakenly assume our religion fits one political spectrum or the next – as though it does not supersede the sphere of politics and man-made constructs all together – is worrying. The attempt to genetically modify Islam with secular strains of thinking that place the primacy of male and male relationships as priority sits in stark opposition to the examples we have from the Sunnah. The many examples where the Prophet ﷺ sought comfort, companionship, humour and support from his wives, and the fact that his marital relationships were built on mutual trust and respect. In reading online Muslim gender discourse, this appears to be an alien concept to a generation who appear to be in a constant impasse with each other.

In addition to this gender symbiosis that Islam unequivocally provides space and precedent for, the idea of Muslim women's rights, based on Islamic tenets and not lies we are being told about our own religion, needs to be reestablished amongst Millennial and Gen Z Muslims in an uplifting, non-patronising way. We need to rewrite the cultural narrative that Muslim women are lollipops and jettison the fable-like narrative of femininity that infantilises us as less than male believers in the eyes of our Creator.

There are countless nuanced debates about how women can better themselves as believers and armour themselves against thinking and practice that is unIslamic in nature –these conversations should also be taking place in Muslim men's spaces. There needs to be more critique from religious and cultural figures which centre men's agency and accountability in this movement which is openly violent and ideologically hostile towards women. The answer to these questions that are generated in the male Muslim community lie exactly there, and as believers in Allāh, Muslim women have to have faith that they will be answered, by the will of Allāh.

...Into the fire

There are of course other cultural shifts germinating online, and which bear upon modern Muslim mothers and their ideals, and naturally they also centre upon the hypergendered roles that are becoming the defining feature of an internet culture gone awry. Chief amongst these is the now burgeoning TradWife trend, and its opposite the Muslimah BossGirl. Concomitant trends, the birth of TradWife came as a direct result of the fourth-wave feminism birthed "girl-boss" era, incepted over fifteen years ago. Defined predominantly in economic terms, girl-boss was a statement of women breaking glass ceilings and being more daring in the work space. TradWife emerged as a counter-culture movement of this expression of femininity, and became highly popularised due to the bordering on ludicrous social media content it gives rise to. Much of which centres on TradWives making the most impossible food and craft items entirely from scratch – be it chewing gum, cereal, paper or crayons – often dressed in formal and flamboyant attire. A bold embodiment of society's maternal fantasies – this breed of TradWife plays on the idea of motherhood as generative and inordinately perfect to a raptured audience of millions. The uniting feature of both movements is that they profess to be iconoclastic, and their appeal is situated in this apparent breaking of rules – though evidently, both are preoccupied with creating newer, more restrictive ones. While they assert that they want to liberate women from man-made impositions, they are adding increasing layers to those punishing social ideals and expectations.

To give one the anodyne social media lowdown of both movements in the Muslim world– one side is the monochrome boldly worded Instagram posts reminding us to go out and be the independent boss woman we are destined to be as believers. The other, eerily saccharine, pastel themed TikToks featuring Muslim women extolling the virtues of serving men. As ever with online movements, the terms of debate begin at such extreme starting points, entrenched in such secular constructs, that we are often forced to pick one of the two sides of a worryingly similar coin – one that defines itself either by or against men, according to traditional Western gender dynamics, and which claims unequivocal religious legitimacy. These movements exemplify how the Muslim woman, and her ability to mother as central to that, becomes the battleground for the ideological wars of our time.

Ironically, both sides of the warring parties adopt male-centric dialogue – our trads accusing the boss girls of dressing according to the male gaze, with the reverse accusations of being a 'pick me'. Effectively both sides appear to be accusing the other of posturing for men. They also both use scripture as the basis for their positions. The sum effect of this eternal back and forth is, that as a community of Muslim women we appear to be stuck in the gear of using men as a yardstick for legitimacy, according to constructs of gender that aren't native to Islamic thought, while being so sadly oblivious to true theology.

What often belies these cyclical and reductive debates, and the polemic values they espouse, is a lack of understanding when it comes to the material reality of Muslim women, religious scripture, or often both. Despite superficial references to economics, and illustrious figures of Islamic history to make their point, both sides often ignore the delicate balance and nuance contained in our situations as respective Muslim women with a love of our Creator, a desire to become wives and often mothers, and the material demands in an increasingly complex world. They are often oblivious to both the merciful discipline contained in Islam, as well as the compassion in it. While we are all well aware of the dangers of reducing our world to restrictive binaries, we are equally just as likely to continue to fall into its ideological and rhetorical trap, by inverting those binaries and using them as definitive guides.

Though the nucleus of this debate remains depressingly similar, TikTok and a digital generation bred on the instance and reactive nature of the algorithm have been kind enough to produce movements that allow us to dress it up in different trends.

Introducing...the TradWife

TradWife is a movement which centres on a kind of cosplay aesthetic, and is now in the full throes of populist limelight and influence. With unsurprising roots, and continuous links, in alt-right movements, it propagates a gender 'traditionalism' that sees the woman as content home-maker, mother and wife, and warns against the entrapments of a modern world in which women eschew domesticity for the shackles of the labour market. It is, paradoxically, a response to an increasingly complex external climate of falling wages, stagnation, and labour insecurity. Almost as if the confusion felt by an increasingly nebulously gendered world is to reset to zero, put on our blindfolds, and feel our way back to seemingly simpler times. Consisting predominantly of young women marketing the idealism of the stay-at-home lifestyle to millions of users, it is a movement that claims universality, and which undoubtedly has a broad and captive audience. However, it speaks exclusively to the situation of women who are in economically secure settings, with no additional demands on their time, interest and capacity – a demographic that is increasingly scarce given the wider economic climate. Think of it as those social media personalities who do unboxing of bags worth more than a few months of the average salary, and how their audience constitutes mainly of women for whom this is unachievable. Many TradWives are selling a certain kind of social and cultural capital, which depends upon a similar economic privilege, to similarly less economically privileged audiences.

This movement has created a validating narrative for some Muslim women who see it as echoing the rights, duties and obligations of women, specifically in relation to the men in their life, as set out in Islam. For others – who have either been victim to or witnessed the subjugation of women in the name of Islam, or for whom this idealised role does not match their own material reality – the TradWife movement and its claim to Islamic validity is justifiably very triggering and worrying. It is also perceived as denigrating to women for whom the brand of domestic bliss is not a possibility.

And herein lies the issue of a naive, social media, aesthetic-powered narrative being attributed to our beautifully substantive religion: it casts a self-righteous finger back at women for whom Allāh has set circumstances different to what are perceived as the 'standard norms'. It is the opposite of our Islamic tradition when we do not account for the situation and context of women such as Mariam, Aasiyah, Aiesha and Khadijah *radi*yallāh*u 'anhum* – for whom being married, a mother and in a loving relationship were not their consistent experiences across time. Allāh has not only given us these examples in our history, but the examples of those Prophets in the Quran who came from homes that did not fit the standard that we ourselves define and attribute to Islam.

In a world where those standards are similarly no longer the norms, this pool of women, who are equal as believers in Islam, and for whom Islam has accommodated, grows – much like the broader female population. Crucially, the negligence of Muslim men in fulfilling their own rights and obligations makes significant contribution to these circumstances, and this is not given the attention and time it currently deserves. All the while, the judgemental call from traditionalist movements, both in TradWife and Red Pill, only grows louder and more alienating against women, some of whom have not been afforded their God-given rights, who require economic independence, and who are beaten down socially due to this. For whom those apparently female duties and obligations are further posed on them as both a punishment and 'cure' for their apparently wayward ways.

The problem with TradWife is it imposes unrealistic standards upon unrealistic standards through its bizarre mix of homemade craft paper and organic beeswax crayons. The wider values and lifestyle this propagates is having real and material impacts on a generation of women who are increasingly sensitive to intractable internet trends and a climate in which social contagion has a dangerous efficacy. The gender cosplay that we see in the infosphere is an often unachievable and unobtainable cookie cutter for gender relations, and Muslim motherhood, in the real world.

Opposing one thing does not mean endorsing its opposite

Undoubtedly, the idea of the committed mother, wife and homemaker certainly isn't worthy of the ridicule it draws, and which is implicit in those that call the TradWife movement out. Nor are these roles necessarily intellectually or spiritually limiting. It is both sneering and wrong to suggest housewives and mothers, and the labour these roles entail, is any less worthy or valuable than other vocations, or that those that are content with it are lesser. In fact, part of the issue is that we are framing both the conflated desire to achieve/work and become a homemaker in economic terms entirely. The need for economic independence in a world where the marriage market is as precarious as it is for Muslim women, is an issue which needs to be separated from the continuing denigration of home making. And creativity, expression, and independence need not always be for economic ends and public consumption.

As we all know, there is no way to quantify the value of the homemaker, and there is undoubtedly a virtue in the role of mother and wife, as prescribed by our Sunnah. But certainly, it is not a universal experience, and not the only path to salvation, and it should not be the sole barometer of faith. As with everything we do as Muslims, it is centring Allāh, rather than man or man-made concepts, that brings the role its virtue and substance. These are both areas that the TradWife movement, as propagated by Muslims, ignores.

Rather, ironically, TradWife as a trend is glorified by those who have become the face of the movement, in as much as it is public-facing and profiteering. The very two things the movement claims are corrupting to women. Therein lies the paradox of a movement birthed by and from capitalism, and the supremacies that underpin it, into a world in which value and meaning is distorted by the endless quest for profit. It's therefore faux 'anti-feminist' in as far as the women making money from it often use the fact they themselves are financially independent because of this grift, as a retort against those that rightly claim the trad life isn't always a viable lifestyle. They are therefore promoting a double standard which protects their right to financial independence at the expense of their audience of women. They also ostensibly propagate a value system which creates a broader sense of meaning and value while reducing their worth to how much they've made from their social media channels. This exposes both how classist and conformist it is as a social media movement, because what they're really trying to say is that, as women of relative comfort and wealth, they have the *choice* of working, while other women shouldn't be afforded the same. TradWife is also framed as a cure for RedPill-ism or Mincel in that many of those that promote it imply that marital respect comes from assuming this hyper-effeminised role. Though this should not be part of the terms of debate, many Mincels in the public eye actually boast about their wives submissiveness while still promoting a harsh, cruel and punitive approach to husbandry.

Once again, these gender debates are entirely reactive and false. Though it doesn't even bear saying, Islamic gender relations were not born from 1950's American sitcoms. Our rights, duties, obligations to each other as man and wife are deep, complex, nuanced and actually very beautiful. The traditionally Western idea that difference cannot be seen outside of a hierarchical structure is counterproductive to relationships which thrive. Equity does not, and should not mean, a clinically black and white sense of equality. As mothers, who have borne the proud physical and emotional battle scars of motherhood, this point is underscored in our very physicality and psyche. There is a humility inherent in being a Muslim husband and father in the same way there is in being a Muslim mother – in understanding yourself as relational beings, a member of creation that is both exceptional and one of many – indeed, exceptional *because* you are one of many – a unique cog in a wider functioning system. There is so much beauty in the humility and empowerment of this realisation.

What this means is, we need to root our ideas of women's rights in the divine rule of Islamic law; this does not mean ignoring or negating other doctrines or claims to female rights, it means using Islam as sole arbiter and not the need to oppose or support any other system. Gender essentialism – the idea that women are inherently one way and men another – has waxed and waned in popularity over the decades. We can't ignore that Allāh has created us differently, this does not need to be a bad thing, however unfashionable it currently seems. Particularly for Muslims with no natural political home, and whose ideological tribalism is often confused by the undulating loyalties of mainstream political movements.

Meet the Muslimah Boss

The Boss Woman, or Muslimah Boss trend, is similarly a much broader movement which has percolated through to Muslim thinking and lifestyle, and which has taken on different iterations of internet trends. In its current neologism, it exposes our messy thinking in both our perception of 'boss' as inherently male and not a naturally 'female' attribute, and the idea of dominance as desirable and aspirational.

It puts emphasis on economic independence, professional achievement and an equally stylised individualism and autonomy. Muslim women keen to reference the social and economic position of Khadijah *radi*allāh*u 'anha* are quick to foreground this as antidote to both the shallow perceptions of TradWife, and our issues as a Muslim community more generally – with respect to the UK, where half of all Muslims live in poverty, this is particularly pertinent.

For Boss Woman and its Muslim iterations, the emphasis remains on wealth and prosperity; achievement as measured by economic productivity – this is distinct from personal, social and spiritual enrichment. It typically promulgates a kind of deficit thinking which positions us as merely consumers who can never quite amass enough 'things'. True to the individualism, and underlying capitalistic ideology, it ignores the fact that systemic issues exist due to society's fixation on a specific kind of 'growth'. Capitalism's inability to value anything outside of financial profit, for example, means that the very value of faith is meaningless, even that faith that references the economic potential of women. Indeed, companies, marketers and economic systems are incentivised to keep us feeling deficient – in faith and otherwise – and in constant 'boss'/economically achieving/"growth" mode. It is symptomatic of a neoliberal, free market world, but rather than eschewing this consumer hungry world like the TradWife claims to, it embraces the apparent glamour of capitalist ideals and all the messy implications that come with it.

Inherently, it is based on the idea that to be more archetypically 'male' is what will grant women greatness. By inverting the gender binary of men as essentially dominant/public facing and women as submissive/domestic dwelling, it only works to buttress the hierarchy that underpins it. It does nothing to interrogate or destabilise it, rather it shallowly embraces ideals we should unequivocally be questioning. In doing so, it endorses a whole host of problematic traits by virtue of their association with a conflated idea of men and dominance and a very specific kind of prosperity alone. What it ignores are the many other forms of growth and enrichment, outside of a capitalist framework, that women, and indeed men, are encouraged to focus on as believers.

Why should women be forced to focus our emotional and intellectual capacity solely as economic productivity? When we know there is both a precedent and need for female Islamic scholarship for example? And why is the only response to this idea which masquerades as 'traditional', for women to be economic agents fuelling an unethical system of greed and consumption? Is this a movement than benefits us or GDP...?

And the false male/female dynamic upon which notions such as the highly effeminised TradWife and the opposing, supposedly more masculine Muslimah Boss are built upon, are themselves flawed. They rest on the duality of mind and body. While historically speaking, men have been associated with the brain and cerebral, high Enlightenment ideals such as intellect and reason, women have been framed as the opposite – manic, emotive and impulsive bodily creatures. While these stereotypes are patently false, and tragically we haven't progressed beyond them culturally, the hierarchy that holds them hostage is equally faulty. The instinctive, intuitive and emotional qualities innate to womanhood and motherhood are valuable and should be celebrated and embraced. The precedent they set, that being a mum is not intellectually stimulating, should also be challenged. It means there is another bar set for women to have to prove their intellectual worth, or once again, to suppress it by. The unfortunate off shoot of this is the derision stay at home mothers face, as though it is an uninformed, anti-intellectual decision. As though it comes from a place of lacking or misunderstanding. This condescending idea that those that choose primarily to mother don't know any better or can't do any better.

An end to duality

Ultimately the duality of Muslimah Boss and TradWife, which define themselves by and against men, both fall massively short of doing Muslim women and our understanding of our roles as believers any real justice. While it would be disingenuous to suggest Islam doesn't recognise a form of gender essentialism, adopting historically and materially false understandings of these gender roles, as emanated through internet trends, reduces our understanding of our illustrious faith. In fact, both movements are reactionary opposites – Muslim Boss Woman a response to a false idea of Islam as 1950's American gender archetypes – and TradWife a doubling down on this false concept.

We have effectively created a binary impression of gender roles, rooted in false cultural and historical ideals, and wrongly attributed it to Islam. This comes from an incorrect and dangerous equivalence which we have all internalised, which we've previously discussed, and which places Islam in opposition to 'modernity'. This falsehood is being projected onto ever more complex real life situations in which men don't appear to always have the economic standing, nor the religious literacy, to allow women to reap the benefits and rights of being a Muslim woman – both inside and outside the home. This is despite the ever loudening calls for women to fulfil a distorted and exaggerated version of the role of women in Islam.

While a frank conversation needs to be had about the ideas concerning femininity, legitimacy, rights and duties of the women in Islam, given the twin-side of this debate featuring masculinity is becoming increasingly disingenuous, we are nowhere near the point where this will be fruitful. Until we redress this sociological imbalance which frames Allāh's Mercy entirely for men, and His punishment and wrath exclusively for women, and creates a Muslim Hive Mind which sees anything propagating women's feelings and rights as akin to heretics, while endorsing male-centric ideologies based on a lurid culture as though it is Islam pure, it seems futile to encourage further discourse.

These encircling and extreme internet debates focus solely on the actions of women, while continuing to prioritise the rights and needs of the man – crucially while leaving Allāh and Islam out altogether. The debate is not whether we are good believers but whether we are good wives or economic agents. While undoubtedly our role as believers will encompass some of the former, it is part of a symbiotic relationship for which men have the perfect role model in the form of our Prophet ﷺ – who showed mercy, kindness, and love to his wives and children. Who partook in the very domestic activities some of the most vocal men in our community deem beneath them – a trait many scholars say grants men honour and respect in the domain of the home. And while women will and have needed to, and drawn satisfaction from, the world of business and commerce, there is simply no spiritual or practical benefit in using this as a defining feature of who we are as Muslim women.

Ultimately, as our lives become more complicated, and gender dynamics need to be given further thought, market forces and internet aesthetics should not be the basis on which we perceive or adopt our sociological roles as either men or women in Islam. They should not be the basis an individual or family creates a template for their set up, as a unit designed entirely to please Allāh.

The gender essentialism Islam does endorse is not one we currently have the language or cultural symbolism in the West to do justice to, due to how heavily fixed we are in the false binary paradigm and the continuing subjugation of Muslim women, ironically, in the name of Islam.

As mentioned, the way we think and talk about Islam is inherently deficient. There is no direct translation for the term '*baraqah*' or '*ihsan*' for example. So when we are gauging our sense of worth – where our energy and output should be directed, as English-speaking Muslims immersed in secular thinking and values, very often we are doing this with a gaping hole in the very metrics by which we asses and enact worth. Very often we begin the conversation omitting the most important, and defining feature of it. Very often it doesn't inhabit a linguistic space in our collective thinking. Our basic notions of our worth, the atomics of how we perceive and communicate them, are subject to wider cultural thinking and values. And work needs to be done to interrogate how we view other terms such as gender essentialism and how that impacts our impressions of them as Muslims, and our ability to engage in meaningful debate concerning them. And this needs to be seen within the context of where this essentialism sits in Islam and what liberty, equality and empowerment really means according to He who created these concepts. While our social roles are shaped differently by shariah as men and women, we are explicitly equal as believers in the sight of Allāh. We stand before Allāh with our actions, and our actions alone. By He who created the very notion of equality, and our ability to perceive and act upon it, we are given the ultimate equality as women in our ultimate purpose – that of worshipper.

And though we might fall into the trap of ignoring

views based on who, or what groups, are espousing them alone (including the Mincel community…) it is important not to fall into the trap of thinking our religion comes from the opposite of what any individual or collective is promoting, as this still constitutes us using them as moral guides. The opposite of Red Pill ideology – or views espoused by male influencers risibly championing 'male rights' – is not Islam, and to use the inverse of what they believe is still to centre them, and their man-made, often half-witted ideology, in our lives. Due to this increasing binary, we have developed a reflex habit of denouncing anything that pertains to 'traditionalism', on the basis it falls under the secular concept of 'traditionalism' alone. Blindly negating it is just as unhelpful as blindly conforming to it. In reality, there are practices that fall within what we might conventionally define as 'traditional' and 'modern' concepts of motherhood that have Islamic weight and credence. Islam, *al-ḥamdulilāh*, is not a reactionary response to anything, it stands on its own feet according to its own purpose, and it's about discovering that without the cultural baggage, nor in sole defiance to it. Between the internet discourse, the cultural expectations, feminist mantra and your own intuition is the role of mother which is based entirely on a Divine mandate, tune out the noise (in both directions) to focus on this alone.

That is, Islamic concepts of gender essentialism aren't necessarily complimentary nor diametrically opposed to 'Western' gender ideals. Islam does not exist as a knee-jerk system nor is it one that needs to appease 'modernity'. It is a totally independent value system. This notion that Muslim men might feel a certain way about a 'dominant' woman is rooted in erroneous ideas regarding gender ideals. Part of masculinity is to feel secure enough to not be intimidated by a woman who might 'challenge' you. If we keep falling back on modern assumptions regarding gender relations, we are doing our faith a disservice.

As a side note, this will involve what has become a dirty word of late, and which is wrongly co-opted by anti-female movements. That is, self-sacrifice. The term itself in many contexts – certainly not all – is a misnomer. In some instances, by learning to compromise you are actually gaining more. The personal, physical, emotional expenses of motherhood are not only banked in a higher plain in the afterlife, but they are also enriching in the material and the 'here'. For so long, the worrying trend of women having to self-sacrifice to their own detriment in some traditionally Muslim cultures has meant that we have sworn off the idea completely. It has also meant we've misunderstood this to be a female trait, rather than a universally Muslim one. Self-discipline and training, compromising on our own wants and needs, is part of what makes us better believers, and the role of motherhood will demand this of you in spades. Embracing this as part of our faith helps us to achieve an aligning of values, reap *barakat* in our actions, and enables us to see and embody our roles in positive, healthy and productive ways.

A possible solution?

For now, maybe we should stop treating marriage entirely like it is an economic exchange, as though it is entirely transactional. Perhaps we would do better to desist from this habit of quoting hadith and Quran, purely to own the opposite gender and promote our own perspective, reducing religious rulings to the logic of competition, only referenced in fractious contexts. Perhaps we should be approaching our scripture with humility and in seeking for ways to become better believers, independently and through our relationships such as marital ones, for the sake of Allāh alone. Not for likes, clout or other forms of kudos, nor the social waves and sensibilities they create.

Perhaps the very network through which we seek public validation – social media – should not be where we form our basic ideas of relationships which require the quiet, inward ponderance required for the *ihsan* and sincerity that makes them successful. Which depend very much on the circumstances we are in and not the broad brush stroke of catch-all, social media content for likes.

Amongst much of the Muslim community there is a damaging reticence concerning essentialism and our roles as men and women, due to the torrid gender landscape we inhabit, and this holds us back from having critical insights, and frank and honest conversations centring the Muslim family and home that would benefit us as a whole. If authenticity in our intentions and faith is the secret ingredient for a healthy relationship, both with ourselves, our spouses, and our children, then should we not be turning inward rather than doing an outward body dive into the cesspit of social approval and recognition? Perhaps we should all be turning unanimously away from spurious internet trends dressed up as Islamic dawah if we really seek the peace and contentment we claim to.

Very often, internet debates are obfuscating and directionless, we run the risk of allowing them to take us further away from our stated aim of closeness to Allāh, as women, when our relationships are mediated with the screen. Perhaps it's time to finally switch some of them off.

POSTSCRIPT

Blessed is He in Whose Hand is the dominion, and He is Able to do all things. Who has created death and life, that He may test you which of you is best in deed.
(Al-Mulk 67:1-2)

Books are meant to conclude with an always well argued, often portentous, multi-paged statement that satisfies its finale-hungry audience. It's the bow that ties all the threads of the argument so neatly into a gratifying conclusion, gifting you a complete perspective and understanding of the subject at hand. So, we can dust off that topic, we've mastered that art, we understand the field of study, existence or being. We've gained enough insight to move on from this topic, even if momentarily.

Any book on mothering that makes such final claims is a farce. And the endeavour to conclude on parenting is even more futile when it comes to Islamic parenting – its most supreme form.

Because parenting is a chemistry, made up of multiple, constantly evolving, temperature sensitive factors; chief amongst them is the living, breathing beast we've just attempted to wrestle through the course of these essays – that is the very environment we parent in. Parenting is also an art form that will draw every part of you in, demanding your creativity, passion and love. It is *ibadah*[28] – itself the greatest act we can engage in and our very nucleus of purpose – an act of worship so uniquely testing and merciful in equal parts. It is entirely natural to us as women whose biology accommodates this very function, and alien to us as social animals with an instinct for individualism. It requires a constant balancing of the innate, natural and socialised elements of our being; those parts that are weather dependent and which change with the tide of age.

Islamic parenting is presupposed on the idea of the parent and child as whole – mind, body and soul. It maps out our existence beyond the materially discernible and outside of our immediate perspective. It acknowledges who we are in the realest sense – believers, and worshippers of Allāh. It has its own rights, responsibilities, obligations and decorum, and its end goal is no

---

[28] Worship

less than Jannah. In this way, it is a great and edifying honour, because it's a position Allāh has put you in as someone with the *taqwā* to see that whole sense of self, and that ultimate human goal, beyond the parameters of what's actually visible. He has set you the ultimate port of call, as someone with all the potential to achieve it, in all its magnanimity. To contribute to the ummah of the Prophet ﷺ, no less.

Islamic parenting bestows upon us that consciousness, the languidly heightened perception of the real and everlasting. It has the ability to grant us access to a new dimension of seeing the world, and afterlife, and finding our place in it. To value *imaan* and *tawakul* as the gold that we sift and pan from the earthly matter of our being.

That lens which Islam rewards us with extends onto our social cartography; how we plot ourselves, as believers, within the wider function of society, and how our parenting impacts this ecosystem. It demands more of us, and our children – a greater sense of social awareness, to understand our worth, and theirs, outside of our limited view of them as ours and ours alone – that stretching of potential and capacity that counters our myopic instinct as humans who may want to trammel ourselves into a restrictive ball of comfort. Islam is a constant reawakening from the slumber of complacency and the sleep walking into social norms for 'normalities' sake alone. It is an active and restless effort at being worthy of the title of slaves of Allāh in that context of bringing and raising other lives. It gives us the tools to enable our children to see themselves in relation to both the Creator and the created, and grants them a unique sense of humility through this social prism. To model to them the quality of *ihsan* in all that we do and commit to.

Islam awards us with a cultural and political consciousness too, which allows us to purify our view of ourselves as those with *ikhlas* (sincerity), and to understand our commitment to justice, truth and fairness. As Muslims we will always be strange, and Allāh sends glad tidings to us in the position we inhabit as strangers in particular. Allāh sends us His blessing in our most isolated role; what greater comfort can we seek, and what better consolation is there for this walk we must make? The political minefield we enter as Muslims – of all colours, and backgrounds – is indicative of the burden of truth that we bear. We are a people of truth, and our honour and integrity is far weightier and worth more than any worldly currency or measure.

These fields – the personal, social, political and cultural – crosscurrent on us as mere souls who are trying to reach the other side, to meet Him in a manner that He may be pleased with, and to enable those we bore, and love the most, to do the same. To take the gut-wrenching beauty He has bestowed upon us through this unique role as this unassuming, monosyllabic title of 'Mum' and to do it a semblance of justice.

And that's what this book is about – that labour. And how those fields of vision; the personal, social, political and cultural, sometimes impair and warp and sometimes bolster and embolden that task of simply getting us all safely to the other side, to meet Him and His messenger with a catalogue of deeds that bear witness for us as those that tried, so constantly, for His sake alone. How the truth stands in stubborn resistance to all that oppose it, and illuminates and elucidates all that compliment it. How those currents wash over us as believers with the ultimate purpose to honour and hold onto that truth until the very end.

This book has attempted to speak to you in the language of motherhood. The motherhood that exists in every layer of our being, our heart, our bones our soul. It sought to speak above the noise of our personal pretensions, the social and digital chatter, the political megaphone and the cultural discourse. Because beneath all those layers of semiotics is something that is coded into our very existence as mothers, to want Islam for our children. Words are only a mere simulation of that language that we speak through our actions, our love and devotion to our children, rooted in our desire to please Him alone. Through the way we shape our very lives to achieve the optimum for their Ākhira[29]. The same language we speak as mothers, is our language as believers, our most acute sense and our most guttural understanding.

Allāh is Merciful in all that He's given us – in how motherhood complements and bulwarks your faith, and how your faith complements and encourages your ability to mother. It is one of the most real human experiences, one that will take you right down to the bone of what it means to exist, and what we are all here for. That kind of realness, in a superficial world, has such great potential, and we've been given the exact tools as Muslims to make the absolute best of it, and the room to do that in a way that is true and forgiving to ourselves. To grant our children themselves this tool, this foresight and clear-eyed perception, as a legacy that will outstand any physical patrimony

---

29 The Hereafter

we can leave them with. Though many of us fixate on leaving our children materially secure, the truth remains, those material provisions are redundant should they not inherit a mindset which sees the world replete with His blessings. No matter what material circumstances we provide our children with, it is redundant if they do not possess the prism with which to see it as a gift from Him and to have contentment with His Decree.

Being a Muslim mum is to know that Islam, if we work hard enough to understand it, gives us the kind of peace that is otherwise invisible to motherhood – the reassurance of an uncompromising truth that we can recline and stretch our full selves into – a limitless resource by which to see and shape the world.

This world, and the lives we carve out for ourselves in it, are a test; they stand as a mirage between us and the true oasis of our purpose. And it's so easy to forget that because of the heady heights and beauties Allāh has granted us in this plain of the here and now. Chief amongst them, our children themselves. If we squint hard enough, we will see how that beauty we see in our children is an actual mirroring of that oasis which Allāh promises us.

It is hard to conclude on the topic of parenting because it is a relationship that really has no conclusion. As always, it is the perennial exception to the rule. Mothering is a constantly evolving element of our being – it is shrouded in a love so strong and lasting its mere presence hints at the existence of afterlife. A love this pure reminds us that there is something beyond our material being. And our deeds live on through our children beyond our own material and worldly conclusion. It is the very notion of our immaterial being as souls, fully symbolised.

As such, there is no real foolproof formula, or manual for Islamic parenting outside of our Quran and Sunnah, unburdened by our own ignorance, bias and shortcomings. The elucidating Quran was sent as guidance, and beyond it there is simply no better guidance – it is our ultimate blue print. And the Noble Prophet ﷺ was sent for the betterment of humanity, and there is simply no better way of life than that which he showed us. This endeavour to follow the Quran and Sunnah, and to foster and hone our children's *imaan* and *taqwā* requires a constant researching, revisiting, repurposing of our intentions and actions. In theory it is beautifully simple, in practice it is as messy as life itself, with the multiple variables that will throw you off course, blur your vision and set obstacles in your path.

When we are constantly seeking to get it right, that mirror through which we see ourselves, and our place in the world is complete and full of truth. As mothers who have been blessed with the ultimate gift – Islam itself – we have the perfect window through which to see ourselves and the world around us. *Inshā'Allāh* we can use it well.

ACKNOWLEDGEMENTS

We begin as always with the praise of Allāh – the Most Beneficial and the Most Merciful, who has bestowed upon us more blessings than we have the ability to conceive and who has gifted us the perfect guide. And with peace and salutations to His Prophet ﷺ who we always strive to emulate. All good in this endeavour, as with everything else, is from Allāh.

Writing a book about motherhood, while simultaneously mothering young children, is a kind of meta I wasn't anticipating. And the acts of writing and mothering hold some eerie similarities – they are both generative, require a kind of focus that grants you a sobering clarity of thought, and are mentally taxing enough to produce a kind of satisfactory, and sometimes tortured, reward. Mothering is such a constant and persistent force in most of our lives, that it breeds a kind of resilience in us that is unmatched – it kind of swallows any hobby, work commitment, or activity we hold in our lives, including writing a book.

Doing both of these rewarding activities in such keen tandem kept the message of the book alive and helped me to live, and convey, a truth that is so specific to us as a tribe of people, particularly as Muslim women, and which can often times feel quite lonely. There are so many people that helped to make this journey less isolated and who have inspired the words in this book.

My own mum, who instilled in me the two ingredients that made it possible to write this book – a love of Allāh and His Messenger, and an obsession with the written word. My dad who always worked so hard for us. My sister who I will never be able to repay in word or deed. And my brothers who are always so resolutely there, thank you.

Hina and Amna – I love you. To my babies Yasmine, Khadijah, Faatimah, Hamd and Aasiyah, for you there are simply no words so I won't even try.

To Rukia and Xara – you both inspire me, may Allāh bless you. To my cousins – too many of you to fit the word count, but so much love for every single one of you nonetheless.

To my oldest friends – Ipek, Shaz, Yath, Sabah, Humera, Mariam and Laura, thank you for every formative memory and current moment, I appreciate you more than I ever say. To those I met through work – Saadia, Shazia, Ruby – and those I met through play (sometimes literally…) – the mums from the North; Hina, Faatimah, Sophie, Tam; aka the OGs, you will always have a special place in my cold and detached heart. Denise, Sidrah, Zainab, Uzma, Saleha, Najibah, Sarah and Jay – always an inspiration, thank you for your presence. To Anna without whom this book would never have been written (you could call it a full circle moment…?) and Nafisa whose sage advice and presence means so much. Anisah who is a legend and taught me so many things that matter.

To those inspiring mums in the East(ish): Tahira, Masuma, Amna, Sabah, Sahra, Sara, Zahida, Hina, Mamoona, Afshan, Mariyam, Saima, Ateeka, Khadijah, Ahsana, Sharifa, Sheba, Radia, Zaynab, Nafisa, Shamaila, Saima, Homa and Adila. Thank you to the beautiful souls in the North West – Nigar, Ayan, Rina, Summera, Sana, Aicha, Noura, Samiah, Safia, Samira, Ramla, Carol, Sedra, Rehma, Sadia, Amreena, Hamdi, Khatera, Fowzia, Zaynab, Sonya, Sarah, Saima, Nailah, Hafsa, Rahela, Mariya, Maheen, Amira and Saida. I've never known a community of women like you.

To Suma for her endless patience and gentleness and to the team at Kube for helping to bring this to life. And Afreen whose talent and skill adorns the cover. To Amaliah – the beautiful sisters and beautiful team without whom we would be bereft of a voice. To Muslim Mamas for being a place of solace for us all. To Sadiya and Everyday Muslim for being amazing. To Imrana for the same! The staff at Haringey public libraries who provide a service many writers would be lost without.

To anyone who's ever read my words and been moved to respond or engage – thank you for your trust.

And to all the Muslim Mothers – for the things we see and the things only Allāh sees – may He bless you all.

ENDNOTES

i   Bridget Brennan, 'Top 10 Things Everyone Should Know About Women Consumers', Forbes, 21 January 2015. Available at: https://www.forbes.com/sites/bridgetbrennan/2015/01/21/top-10-things-everyone-should-know-about-women-consumers/

ii   Algerian boxer Imane Khelif becomes target of Olympics gender row, Al Jazeera, 2 August 2024. Available at: https://www.aljazeera.com/news/2024/8/2/algerian-boxer-imane-khelif-becomes-target-of-gender-row-at-olympics

iii   John Berger, Ways of Seeing, (London, England: Penguin Classics, 2008)

iv   Laura Pritschet, Caitlyn M. Taylor, Daniela Cossio et al, 'Neuroanatomical changes observed over the course of a human pregnancy', *Nature Neuroscience*, 29th July 2024. Available at: https://doi.org/10.1038/s41593-024-01741-0

v   Jeffrey Jensen Arnett 'Getting Better All the Time: Trends in Risk Behavior Among American Adolescents Since 1990', *Archives of Scientific Psychology*, 2018. Available at: https://doi.org/10.1037/arc0000046

vi   OECD, *Society at a Glance 2024: OECD Social Indicators* (Paris: OECD Publishing, 2024). Available at: https://doi.org/10.1787/918d8db3-en

vii   Reid Kikuo Johnson, 'A Mother's Work', cover art, *The New Yorker*, 2 September 2024. Available at: https://www.newyorker.com/culture/cover-story/cover-story-2024-09-09

viii 'Parenting in America Today: A Survey Report', *Pew Research Center* , January 2023. Available at: https://www.pewresearch.org/social-trends/2023/01/24/parenting-in-america-today/

ix Mike Allen, 'Sean Parker unloads on Facebook: 'God only knows what it's doing to our children's brains'.' *Axios*, *9 November 2017*. Available at: https://www.axios.com/2017/12/15/sean-parker-unloads-on-facebookgod-only-knows-what-its-doing-to-our-childrens-brains-1513306792

x Ted Gioia, 'The State of the Culture', *The Honest Broker*, 18 February 2024. Available at: https://www.honest-broker.com/p/the-state-of-the-culture-2024

xi Ibid

xii Christopher Nguyen, 'Value Capture', *Journal of Ethics and Social Philosophy* May 2024. Available at: https://doi.org/10.26556/jesp.v27i3.3048

xiii Whitney Crenna-Jennings, 'Young people's mental and emotional health: Trajectories and drivers in childhood and adolescence', *The Education Policy Institute (EPI) and The Prince's Trust*, January 2021.Available at: https://epi.org.uk/wp-content/uploads/2021/01/EPI-PT_Young-people%E2%80%99s-wellbeing_Jan2021.pdf

xiv Christopher St. Aubin and Jake Liedke, 'Social Media and News Fact Sheet', *Pews Research Centre*, 15 November 2023. Available at:https://www.pewresearch.org/journalism/fact-sheet/social-media-and-news-fact-sheet/

xv Right Response Team, 'The Far Right and the Southport Riot: What We Know So Far', *Hope Not Hate*, , 31 July 2024. Available at: https://hopenothate.org.uk/2024/07/31/the-far-right-and-the-southport-riot-what-we-know-so-far/

xvi Massoumi Narzanin, Tom Mills and David Miller, *'What is Islamophobia? Racism, Social Movements and the State'*, (London: Pluto Press, 2017).

xvii Nadya Ali and Ben Whitham, 'The Unbearable Anxiety of being: Ideological fantasies of British Muslims beyond the politics of security', , 2018, *Sage Publications*

xviii Charles Hymas and Ben Farmer, 'Exclusive: Half of UK's imported Covid-19 infections in June are from Pakistan', *Telegraph*, 26 June 2020. Available at: https://www.telegraph.co.uk/news/2020/06/26/exclusive-half-uks-imported-june-covid-19-infections-pakistan/

xix Libération, @libe, 11 March 2024, *Ramadan à Gaza* [Tweet/X Post], X formerly known as Twitter https://x.com/libe/status/1767067934327742746?s=46

xx Lena Schega, 'Israel-Palestine and the demise of journalism', *The Glasgow Guardian*, 16 February 2024. Available at: https://glasgowguardian.co.uk/2024/02/16/israel-palestine-and-the-demise-of-journalism/

xxi Nadine White, 'Peer accused of Islamophobia after claiming 'radicals will take us over through power of the womb'', *The Independent*, 30 July 2024. Available at: https://www.independent.co.uk/news/uk/politics/lord-pearson-rannoch-speech-islamophobia-b2587610.html

xxii Shadi Hamid, 'The role of Islam in European populism: How refugee flows and fear of Muslims drive right-wing support,' *Brookings Institution*, February 2019. Available at: https://www.brookings.edu/articles/the-role-of-islam-in-european-populism-how-refugee-flows-and-fear-of-muslims-drive-right-wing-support/

xxiii Barbara Perry , 'Social Identities (2013): Gendered Islamophobia: hate crime against Muslim women',*Social Identities: Journal for the Study of Race, Nation and Culture, DOI*. Available at: http://dx.doi.org/10.1080/13504630.2013.864467

xxiv Marcus Ryder, 'The Sesame Street Effect: Why UK Broadcasters are Losing Their Black and Asian Audiences', *The Generation Game: Can the BBC Win Over Today's Young Audiences* (Bite-Sized Books, 2020)

xxv Ibid

xxvi BBC News, 'Shamima Begum: Family of pregnant IS teen plead for return', *BBC News*, 16 February 2019. Available at: https://www.bbc.com/news/uk-47260916

xxvii Josh Baker, 'Shamima Begum: Spy for Canada smuggled schoolgirl to Syria', *BBC News*, 31August 2022. Available at: https://www.bbc.com/news/uk-62726954

xxviii Talk, @TalkTV, 15th August 2024, *"I don't think it's right to make political points with children."* Isabelle Oakeshott says it's "absolutely grotesque" that a 15-year-old became the first person charged with an offence of "riot" @IsabelOakeshott | @ThatAlexWoman [Tweet/X Post], X formerly known as Twitter https://x.com/talktv/status/1824153973885956545?s=46

xxix Jacob Dirnhuber, 'Shamima Begum's mum fears jihadi bride daughter will 'brainwash' grandchild', *The Sun*, 16 July 2020. Available at: https://www.thesun.co.uk/news/8497417/shamima-begum-mum-jihadi-bride-daughter-brainwash-grandchild/

xxx David Cameron, 'We won't let women be second class citizens', *The Times*, 18 January 2016. Available at: https://www.thetimes.com/article/we-wont-let-women-be-second-class-citizens-brh07l6jttb

xxxi BBC News, 'Macron warning on stigmatising Muslims amid France veil row', *BBC News*, 17 October, 2019. Available at: https://www.bbc.com/news/world-europe-50079997

xxxii *Good Morning Britain*, 'Shamima Begum Says She'd 'Rather Die' Than Return to ISIS as She Seeks Forgiveness', *YouTube Channel*, 15th September 2021. Available at: https://www.youtube.com/watch?v=oYfjM_nI4JE

xxxiii Marcus Ryder, 'The Sesame Street Effect: Why UK Broadcasters are Losing Their Black and Asian Audiences', *The Generation Game: Can the BBC Win Over Today's Young Audiences* (Bite-Sized Books, 2020)

xxxiv Tasmiha Khan, 'New reporting project will explore experiences of Muslim women during childbirth in America',

, *USC, Center for Health Journalism*, December 2023. Available at: https://centerforhealthjournalism.org/our-work/insights/new-reporting-project-will-explore-experiences-muslim-women-during-childbirth

xxxv   Marian Knight, Kathryn Bunch and Derek Tuffnell, et al, 'Saving Lives, Improving Mothers' Care Lessons learned to inform maternity care from the UK and Ireland Confidential Enquiries into Maternal Deaths and Morbidity 2017-19', *Maternal, Newborn and Infant Clinical Outcome Review Programme, MBRRACE-UK*, November 2021. Available at: https://www.npeu.ox.ac.uk/assets/downloads/mbrrace-uk/reports/maternal-report-2021/MBRRACE-UK_Maternal_Report_2021_-_FINAL_-_WEB_VERSION.pdf

xxxvi   Shaista Gohir OBE, 'INVISIBLE Maternity Experiences of Muslim Women from Racialised Minority Communities', *Muslim Women's Network UK*, July 2022. Available at: https://www.mwnuk.co.uk//go_files/resources/maternity_report_120722.pdf

xxxvii   Ibid

xxxviii   Mareike Schomerus, Sherine El Taraboulsi–McCarthy, Jassi Sandhar, 'Countering violent extremism (Topic Guide)', *GSDRC, University of Birmingham*, March 2017. Available at: https://assets.publishing.service.gov.uk/media/58e64e6140f0b606e30000fb/CVE.pdf

xxxix   Sam Francis, 'Row over Tory MP's Allāhu Akbar arrest call', *BBC News*, 7 August 2024. Available at: https://www.bbc.com/news/articles/clynl828yp0o

xl   *The Telegraph*, "Protesters chant 'Allāhu Akbar' in Rochdale after police officer 'stamps on man's head'" , *You Tube Channel*, July 2024. Available at: https://www.youtube.com/watch?v=4vTbg6jUKB8&rco=1

xli   Professor John Holmwood and Dr Layla Aitlhadj, 'The People's Review of Prevent', *Prevent Watch*, , February 2022. Available at: https://peoplesreviewofprevent.org/prop-report/

xlii Ibid

xliii Dr Tarek Younis, 'The UK's PREVENT policy would not prevent white supremacist attacks like Christchurch – it's part of the problem', *Media Diversified*, 1 April 2019. Available at : https://mediadiversified.org/2019/04/01/the-uks-prevent-policy-would-not-prevent-white-supremacist-attacks-like-christchurch-its-part-of-the-problem/

xliv Branwen Jeffreys and Jess Warren, 'Michaela School: Muslim student loses prayer ban challenge', *BBC News*, , 16 April 2024. Available at: https://www.bbc.com/news/uk-england-london-68731366

xlv John Holmwood and Therese O'Toole, *Countering Extremism in British Schools? The Truth About the Birmingham Trojan Horse Affair* (Policy Press and Bristol University Press, November 2017).

xlvi Professor John Holmwood and Dr Layla Aitlhadj, 'The People's Review of Prevent', *Prevent Watch*, , February 2022. Available at: https://peoplesreviewofprevent.org/prop-report/

xlvii Ibid

xlviii Ted Gioia, 'How to Know If You're Living in a Doom Loop', *The Honest Broker*, 02 August 2024. Available at: https://www.honest-broker.com/p/how-to-know-if-youre-living-in-a?utm_source=substack&publication_id